Assisted Reproductive Technologies in the Third Phase

Fertility, Reproduction and Sexuality

General Editors:

Soraya Tremayne, Founding Director, Fertility and Reproduction Studies Group and Research Associate, Institute of Social and Cultural Anthropology, University of Oxford.
Marcia C. Inhorn, William K. Lanman, Jr., Professor of Anthropology and International Affairs, Yale University.
Philip Kreager, Director, Fertility and Reproduction Studies Group, and Research Associate, Institute of Social and Cultural Anthropology and Institute of Human Sciences, University of Oxford.

Volume 1
Managing Reproductive Life: Cross-Cultural Themes in Fertility & Sexuality
Edited by Soraya Tremayne

Volume 2
Modern Babylon? Prostituting Children in Thailand
Heather Montgomery

Volume 3
Reproductive Agency, Medicine and the State: Cultural Transformations in Childbearing
Edited by Maya Unnithan-Kumar

Volume 4
A New Look at Thai AIDS: Perspectives from the Margin
Graham Fordham

Volume 5
Breast Feeding and Sexuality: Behaviour, Beliefs & Taboos among the Gogo Mothers in Tanzania
Mara Mabilia

Volume 6
Ageing without Children: European and Asian Perspectives on Elderly Access to Support Networks
Edited by Philip Kreager & Elisabeth Schröder-Butterfill

Volume 7
Nameless Relations: Anonymity, Melanesia and Reproductive Gift Exchange between British Ova Donors and Recipients
Monica Konrad

Volume 8
Population, Reproduction and Fertility in Melanesia
Edited by Stanley J. Ulijaszek

Volume 9
Conceiving Kinship: Assisted Conception, Procreation and Family in Southern Europe
Monica M. E. Bonaccorso

Volume 10
Where There is No Midwife: Birth and Loss in Rural India
Sarah Pinto

Volume 11
Reproductive Disruptions: Gender, Technology, and Biopolitics in the New Millennium
Edited by Marcia C. Inhorn

Volume 12
Reconceiving the Second Sex: Men, Masculinity, and Reproduction
Edited by Marcia C. Inhorn, Tine Tjørnhøj-Thomsen, Helene Goldberg and Maruska la Cour Mosegaard

Volume 13
Transgressive Sex: Subversion and Control in Erotic Encounters
Edited by Hastings Donnan and Fiona Magowan

Volume 14
European Kinship in the Age of Biotechnology
Edited by Jeanette Edwards and Carles Salazar

Volume 15
Kinship and Beyond: The Genealogical Model Reconsidered
Edited by Sandra Bamford and James Leach

Volume 16
Islam and New Kinship: Reproductive Technology and the Shariah in Lebanon
Morgan Clarke

Volume 17
Childbirth, Midwifery and Concepts of Time
Edited by Christine McCourt

Volume 18
Assisting Reproduction, Testing Genes: Global Encounters with the New Biotechnologies
Edited by Daphna Birenbaum-Carmeli and Marcia C. Inhorn

Volume 19
Kin, Gene, Community: Reproductive Technologies among Jewish Israelis
Edited by Daphna Birenbaum-Carmeli and Yoram S. Carmeli

Volume 20
Abortion in Asia: Local Dilemmas, Global Politics
Edited by Andrea Whittaker

Volume 21
Unsafe Motherhood: Mayan Maternal Mortality and Subjectivity in Post-War Guatemala
Nicole S. Berry

Volume 22
Fatness and the Maternal Body: Women's Experiences of Corporeality and the Shaping of Social Policy
Edited by Maya Unnithan-Kumar and Soraya Tremayne

Volume 23
Islam and Assisted Reproductive Technologies: Sunni and Shia Perspectives
Edited by Marcia C. Inhorn and Soraya Tremayne

Volume 24
Militant Lactivism? Attachment Parenting and Intensive Motherhood in the UK and France
Charlotte Faircloth

Volume 25
Pregnancy in Practice: Expectation and Experience in the Contemporary US
Sallie Han

Volume 26
Nighttime Breastfeeding: An American Cultural Dilemma
Cecília Tomori

Volume 27
Globalized Fatherhood
Edited by Marcia C. Inhorn, Wendy Chavkin and José-Alberto Navarro

Volume 28
Cousin Marriages: Between Tradition, Genetic Risk and Cultural Change
Edited by Alison Shaw and Aviad Raz

Volume 29
Achieving Procreation: Childlessness and IVF in Turkey
Merve Demircioğlu Göknar

Volume 30
Thai in Vitro: Gender, Culture and Assisted Reproduction
Andrea Whittaker

Volume 31
Assisted Reproductive Technologies in the Third Phase: Global Encounters and Emerging Moral Worlds
Edited by Kate Hampshire and Bob Simpson

ASSISTED REPRODUCTIVE TECHNOLOGIES IN THE THIRD PHASE

Global Encounters and Emerging Moral Worlds

Edited by Kate Hampshire and Bob Simpson

berghahn
NEW YORK • OXFORD
www.berghahnbooks.com

First published in 2015 by
Berghahn Books
www.BerghahnBooks.com

Library of Congress Cataloging-in-Publication Data
Assisted reproductive technologies in the third phase: global encounters and emerging moral worlds / edited by Kate Hampshire and Bob Simpson.
pages cm
Includes bibliographical references and index.
ISBN 978-1-78238-807-4 (hardback: alk. paper) -- ISBN 978-1-78238-808-1 (ebook)
1. Human reproductive technology--Moral and ethical aspects. 2. Globalization--Social aspects. 3. Human reproductive technology--Developing countries. 4. Human embryo--Transplantation. I. Hampshire, Kate. II. Simpson, Bob, 1956-
RG133.5.A87 2015
618.1'7806--dc23

2015002061

British Library Cataloguing in Publication Data
A catalogue record for this book is available from the British Library.

Printed on acid-free paper

ISBN 978-1-78238-807-4 (hardback)
ISBN 978-1-78238-808-1 (ebook)

CONTENTS

Introduction

Assisted Reproductive Technologies

A Third Phase?

Bob Simpson and Kate Hampshire

The story of assisted reproductive technologies (ARTs) is a remarkable one.[1] That sperm and ova can be taken from a man and a woman, brought together in a petri dish to achieve conception and then implanted back into the womb of a woman where the early stage embryo will come to term, was a technical feat that was to have profound consequences. With the birth of Louise Brown in 1978 the era of the 'test-tube baby' had begun, and with it the emergence of a powerful confluence of biomedical, social and economic interests. Coupling the desires of those who are involuntarily childless with medical and pharmaceutical interests has led to an inexorable rise in the visibility and availability of ART services. Moreover, it has propelled their assimilation and acceptance into everyday worlds of family formation; the exceptional has become ordinary, or at least as ordinary as any human conception can ever be. It was reported at the European Society of Human Reproduction and Embryology's annual meeting in Istanbul in 2012 that some five million babies had been born around the world with the aid of ARTs (ESHRE 2012; Franklin 2012).

Echoing an earlier prediction made by Paul Rabinow in relation to the new genetics, the power of ARTs to reshape ideas of identity and relationality is such because developments of this kind 'will be embedded throughout the social fabric at the micro-level' (Rabinow 1996: 100). But the diffusion of ARTs has other consequences. Beyond the elementary assistance offered to a husband and wife using their own gametes to achieve conception are a plethora of other possibilities. Third-party provision of sperm, ova or fertilised embryos used with techniques such as in vitro fertilisation (IVF), intra-uterine insemination (IUI) and intra-cytoplasmic sperm injection (ICSI) bring novel relational possibilities. For example, mothers may donate eggs to their daughters thereby creating children who are both their 'grandchildren' and 'children' at the same time, as in the Melanie Boivin case.[2] Male couples may employ the services of surrogates and egg donors to produce offspring that are biologically, socially and economically their own, as in the case of Tony Barlow and Barry Drewitt.[3] Further possibilities are added given that gametes and embryos can be cryopreserved for use at some point in the future, enabling posthumous conception to take place, as in the case of Diane Blood.[4] These combinations take reproduction and parenthood beyond existing norms and expectations. As such, they pose significant challenges to prevailing ethical, legal and religious orthodoxies. Not least of these challenges is the potential for commoditisation of gametes and embryos, which threatens to dislodge these substances from their positions within existing schemes of meaning and value.

The anthropological literature on ARTs in the UK and the US has provided groundbreaking accounts of these encounters between novelty and convention in the realms of kinship, family and reproduction (Strathern 1992a, 1992b; Edwards 1993; Franklin 1997; Thompson 2005). These accounts described what we might think of ARTs in their first phase, a period approximating the 1980s and 1990s, in which extra-corporeal conception became available to a relatively small number of people in Europe, North America and the Middle East. Services were available, but mostly in the private sector for those able to pay substantial sums for their own treatment.

The second phase of ARTs, from the late 1990s on, saw the spread of IVF across the globe, with take up mostly by elites through private sector provision. A 'Euro-American' perspective on ARTs was soon augmented by accounts of IVF from a wider range of countries. Accounts of IVF cultures around the world include Israel (Kahn 2000; Nahman 2013), Italy (Bonnacorso-Rothe 2009), Spain (Orobitg and Salasar 2005), China (Handwerker 2002), Ecuador (Roberts 2006), Egypt (Inhorn 1994a),

Lebanon (Clarke and Inhorn 2011), Iran (Tremayne 2006, 2009), India (Bharadwaj 2008) and Sri Lanka (Simpson 2001a, 2004a, 2004b, 2004c, 2005). These ethnographies illuminate the distinctive forms that parenthood and relationality take when ARTs become available in diverse cultural settings. With the exception of Israel, where publicly funded fertility services sit within a wider policy of state-supported pro-natalism, access to ARTs in the countries listed above is mostly the preserve of those who can afford to pay for services. The commercial orientation of ART provision has rendered these services an important site of inequality in terms of class, race, ethnicity and gender, and as such are an important contributor to what Colen earlier identified as 'reproductive stratification' (Colen 1986). To date then, the study of ARTs in the second phase has mostly focused on a relatively small number of global elites accessing services commercially, either in their own countries or following travel abroad (Ginsberg and Rapp 1995; Culley et al. 2011). Set against the global burden of infertility, one could argue that this focus has produced a disproportional effect. ARTs, accessed by the few, have influenced the reproductive desires of the many, both as an icon of technologically assisted reproduction and as a source of powerful rhetoric about medicalised reproduction. Media coverage plays a major part in this process, continuing to 'shape reproductive expectation and desires, particularly when reproductive "miracles" become the focus of media frenzy' (Inhorn and Van Balen 2002: 5).

Yet, this picture is changing, and it is aspects of this change that we explore in this volume. Although at an early stage, it appears that delivery of ARTs is spreading beyond the private sector, both in first world and third world settings, as these technologies become increasingly recognised as part of a standard repertoire of medical assistance for infertility. Increasing accessibility and acceptability mean that far from being rare and exceptional, ARTs are, for an ever-widening constituency, becoming part of routine expectation. This we refer to as ARTs in their third phase – an extension of access and availability that further integrates ARTs into infertility treatment across the globe. We have identified two stepping-off points for our interest in this important phase in the development of ARTs. The first concerns publicly funded access to ARTs in the UK, and the second, the move to recognise infertility as a disease (rather than mere misfortune) and to mobilise treatments to address it as such in developing world settings.

Stepping-Off Point One: Publicly Funded Access to ARTs in the UK

In recent decades, infertility and its consequences have become increasingly visible in the UK. In the 1980s it was estimated that one in six British couples who wished to have children were unable to do so (Hull, Galzener and Kelly 1985). More recent estimates have resulted in predictions of an 'infertility time bomb', with as many as one in three couples having difficulty conceiving.[5] Amongst the growing list of contributory factors are later age of first pregnancy (often blurring the distinction between voluntary and involuntary childlessness), an increase in sexually transmitted diseases, childhood obesity and a consequent rise of conditions such as polycystic ovary syndrome. Involuntary childlessness is a cause of major distress, bringing significant physical, emotional and social consequences. Failing to conceive when there is an explicit desire to do so is also a condition with which others easily identify, and is often construed in terms of desperation and tragedy (Franklin 1997). Furthermore, a widespread response to this condition is a willingness to go to considerable physical, emotional and economic lengths to achieve a pregnancy that will result in a child that might be thought of in some way as one's own.

With the development of ARTs there has been a growing recognition that infertility is not merely an unfortunate personal circumstance but a recognised condition for which a growing range of treatment options exist and, furthermore, that policies should be formulated and resources committed to its alleviation.[6] As a consequence, in the UK over the last twenty years, the use of assisted reproductive technologies has gone from being something that was exceptional and rare to being relatively commonplace, with points of access available across a range of National Health Service (NHS) and private clinics.[7] To this end, in 2004 the UK's National Institute of Clinical Excellence (NICE) issued guidelines for NHS hospitals on the provision of fertility treatments. If certain conditions were met then patients could expect up to three cycles of IVF to be provided and funded by the state.[8]

This move can be seen as part of a wider pan-European trend to support infertility services through the public purse. A recent survey by the European Society of Human Reproduction and Embryology (ESHRE) reported that 1,051 clinics operating in thirty-six European countries (three more than in 2007) reported 532,260 treatment cycles, representing a 7.9 per cent increase in the activity since 2007 (Ferraretti et al. 2012). Furthermore, monitoring by ESHRE suggests that more ART cycles per million of population were performed in countries where public funding was more easily available. For example, in Belgium and Denmark, where state funding is generous, 2,479 and 2,450 ART cycles per million of population were recorded in 2008. In Germany, Italy and UK, where state funding is less generous, the number of cycles per million were 801, 807 and 825 respectively. These figures have led health economist Mark Connelly to suggest that state policies for the funding of fertility treatment through public reimbursement has a direct influence on national birth rates.[9] At a time when fertility rates have declined below replacement levels across Europe, these findings have important consequences, suggesting that ARTs may have a role to play in stabilising population ageing/decline by addressing unmet need for fertility treatment.

Our interest in the specifics of these broader demographics of infertility began with an ESRC-funded project which set out to investigate the ways in which British Pakistani Muslims understand and negotiate involuntary childlessness with particular reference to the solutions offered by the ARTs.[10] In this research, we considered how the explicit intention to provide greater access to infertility treatments was received and acted upon by ethnic minority groups, and specifically those from the Pakistani Muslim community. As a culturally distinct community, Pakistanis are typically characterised as conservative in their patterns of kinship and community, family formation and reproductive behaviour, and their ideas about the place of children in the family (Berthoud 2005; Thapan 2005). Most Pakistanis also have a strong relationship with Islam as a guide to action generally, but particularly when faced with adversity. We were interested to learn more about the reproductive problems experienced by couples from this community, their ways of dealing with them and the issues faced by service providers in ensuring equal and appropriate access to treatments.

The research was carried out at a time when, despite a small upturn, low and late fertility looked set to be sustained in the UK, along with the rest of Europe (Goldstein, Sobotka and Jasilioniene 2009). However, along with British Bangladeshis, British Pakistanis continue to have much higher fertility rates than the UK national average: close to three children per woman (Coleman and Dubuq 2010). British Pakistanis in particular have low levels of childlessness and higher progression to third and higher-order births than the general British population (Modood 1997; Penn and Lambert 2002; Sobotka 2008). Maintenance of high fertility is often attributed to a strongly pro-natalist ideology and normative pressures to bear children (although, as we show elsewhere, this is not necessarily the case uniformly [Hampshire, Blell and Simpson 2012a]). However, high fertility at a population level does not equate with uniform fertility, and rates of infertility among the UK's South Asian populations also appear to be elevated, due in part to a relatively high prevalence of polycystic ovary syndrome-related infertility (Rodin et al. 1998). Where pro-natalism is strong, the consequences of impaired or delayed fertility can be all the greater for individuals who experience reproductive disruption (Inhorn 2003c; Hampshire, Blell and Simpson 2012b). For couples who find themselves in this situation, the suffering that ensues can be acute. As we go on to demonstrate, the quest for resolution is not merely biomedical but connects with a tangle of interests that are cultural, moral and economic.

Stepping-Off Point Two: ARTs in Developing World Contexts

The second stepping-off point is, on the face of it, a long way from the first. At the workshop held at the end of our 'Pakistani Muslims and ARTs' project, it was apparent from the contributions of Frank Van Balen, Johanne Sundby and Willem Ombelet regarding reproductive technologies in lower-income countries that there were important connections. These presentations led us to think more carefully about the availability of ARTs in the economically developing world and a growing recognition of 'the reproductive desires and dilemmas of infertile women and men living outside the West' (Inhorn and Van Balen 2002: 6; see also Vayena et al. 2009). The discussions that followed, particularly with the UK fertility consultants present, suggested that many of the problems of infertility and likely solutions in resource-poor communities were ones that had resonances in their own practices in the UK. Suffice it to say that similar challenges and issues emerged in both contexts, despite some very different drivers for ARTs operating in better-resourced settings in the global north. A key difference is the exceptionally high levels of infertility found in many resource-poor settings (Inhorn 2009). Fertility impairment is in turn caused by the prevalence of sexually transmitted infections, high numbers of unsafe abortions and frequent postpartum pelvic infections, all of which contribute to high rates of tubal factor infertility that are two to four times higher than in other parts of the world (ibid.). Many of the conditions prevalent in the developing world could be avoided through improved public health measures. However, once these conditions are in place they are difficult to treat; prevention is infinitely better than cure. ARTs offer one of the few solutions should fertility be disrupted by one of these conditions, and much work has been carried out recently into the development of low-cost treatments (Ombelet and Campo 2007; also see this volume). The issue of low-cost IVF was of particular interest to the UK consultants attending the workshop when considering access to services in the UK.

An important event in recognising the importance of affordable access to fertility treatments in resource-poor settings was the conference organised by the ESHRE Special Task Force on Infertility in Developing Countries, held in 2008 in Arusha, Tanzania (Ombelet and Van Balen 2010; Ombelet, this volume). This multidisciplinary conference brought together representatives of the most significant organisations operating in the infertility field, along with practitioners and academics. One of the outcomes of the meeting was the setting up of a series of pilot studies in which affordable treatments for infertility were trialled in Genk, Belgium, with the eventual aim of introducing these into resource-poor areas (Johnson, Cohen and Grudszinskas 2014; Ombelet 2014; Van Blerkon et al. 2014).

The project of providing assistance to those experiencing reproductive disruption in developing-world settings has elicited concerns and criticism throughout its history. It is argued that ARTs are not a priority in resource-poor settings, where population pressures are high and there is likely to be poor medical infrastructure, regulation and quality control (Macklin 1995; Okonofua 1996; Vayena et al. 2009). Combined with the low success rate of ARTs, there is likely to be major disappointment for those facing infertility, given that expectations will be high and results sparse (Edouard and Olatunbosun 1997). Finally, feminist concerns identify a continuing focus on women's procreative roles in ARTs as symptomatic of an abiding patriarchy and the exploitation and appropriation of women's bodies (Rapp 2001). Recognition of the plight of those with reproductive difficulties has not entirely escaped international policy. The International Conference on Population and Development (ICPD) held in Cairo led to United Nations Programme of Action 1995, which recognised 'the rights of men and women to choose the number, timing and spacing of their children by calling for reproductive health programmes to include the prevention and appropriate treatment of infertility' (ICPD 1994; also see Nachtigall 2006: 871). However, as Ombelet and others in this volume suggest, infertility remains something of a Cinderella issue, which has failed to grab the attention of major donors or achieve prominence in the Millennium Development Goals-driven global health agenda.

Three Themes in the Third Phase of ARTs

Both of the above stepping-off points suggest the beginning of an opening up of ARTs to new constituencies in terms of ethnicity, geography, education and class. With this widening of access, reproductive 'assistance' is summoned in very diverse settings in terms of lay beliefs about procreation, body and relationships. Here we see the biomedical responses to frustrated reproductive desire framed within evermore diverse notions of family, kin and community, and shaped by distinct configurations of morals and values. In this respect, we might simply record that ARTs become even further embedded in day-to-day life. However, we would like to draw attention to three themes that provide significant points of overlap between the two very different stepping-off points identified above. These are the fertility–infertility dialectic, globalisation, and a form of moral pioneering that entails what we have termed 'the bricolage of bioethics'.

The Fertility–Infertility Dialectic

A key feature of many of the populations that are being reached in a third phase of ARTs is that they already appear to have high levels of fertility. This may well be true at a population level but, for those who have the misfortune to encounter 'barrenness amid plenty' (Van Balen and Gerrits 2001), the consequences of infertility can be seriously amplified by what Inhorn has referred to as the fertility–infertility dialectic: a situation in which the prevalence of infertility is often greatest where fertility is the highest (Inhorn 1996, 2003b, 2003c, 2007b). The problem is further compounded by the fact that many of the steps taken to increase fertility are the very things that might impair it (for example, unprotected sex and sex with multiple partners, both of which increase the likelihood of infertility linked with sexually transmitted infection). Where there are strong expectations surrounding fertility, the occurrence of infertility can be particularly catastrophic, leading couples into a relentless 'quest for conception' (Inhorn 2003c: 1838). Furthermore, experiences of infertility may be structured by gender, social class, age and ethnicity, which can interact to compound the suffering and disempowerment of childless women, particularly those with few other options for gaining social status and security (Inhorn 1996: 2; Riessman 2000, 2002).

A perception that emerges from this paradox in populations with relatively high fertility (including the UK Pakistani Muslim context and many other contexts, particularly in the 'developing world') concerns the issue of fertility control in populations that are already seen as over-producing. The attribution of 'hyper-fertility' to some populations means that infertility is either ignored or even welcomed by policymakers as a 'solution' to overpopulation (Van Balen and Inhorn 2002; Greil, Slauson-Blevins and McQuillan 2010; Ombelet this volume). The use of ARTs in these contexts is also seen as an unhelpful distraction from other more pressing health priorities that may afflict such communities, such as high rates of maternal and child mortality, and a heavy burden of infectious diseases like HIV, TB and Malaria (Macklin 1995; Okonofua 1996): 'infertility is relatively unimportant in low-resource settings where fatal and contagious diseases remain uncontrolled' (Vayena et al. 2002: 13; also see Van Zandvoort, de Koning and Gerrits 2001). Measures aimed at increasing fertility in such settings might appear to be counter-intuitive when population control and lack of effective contraception pose serious challenges to public health and well-being.

Such views are further reinforced in the UK when set against demographic concerns about the rates at which different groups reproduce.[11] Anxieties have recently been further raised by suggestions that there is a close link between religion, ethnicity and fertility, such that those who are most strongly affiliated to a religious way of life are also more likely to have the biggest families – secularists it would seem do not reproduce terribly well (Kaufman 2010). In other words, 'society', and prevailing views of fertility therein, provide an important context within which to situate discussions about infertility among ethnic minority communities in Western countries, as well as among the poor in developing-world ones.

Yet, in both these contexts, it is clear that what is the subject of erasure when viewed at the level of populations and demography is all too visible when viewed at the level of families and individuals (Vayena, Rowe and Peterson 2002). In otherwise 'high-fertility' settings, the social, psychological and economic impacts of infertility impacts are both significant and disproportionate (Gerrits 1997; Bhatti, Fikree and Khan 1999; Riessman 2000; Bharadwaj 2003; Van Balen and Bos 2009; Nahar 2010). In this volume we explore the finer grain of these contradictions and the ways in which ARTs become woven into prevailing ideas about fertility and infertility in settings that fall outside of 'two-will-do' norms and practices.

Reproductive Technologies as Global Form

In December 2008, seventy-two clinicians, scientists, epidemiologists and social scientists gathered together at the World Health Organization (WHO) headquarters in Geneva, Switzerland, to work out an agreed vocabulary to be deployed worldwide when using ARTs (Zegers-Hochschild et al. 2009). The driver for this initiative was the need to 'benchmark' and 'standardise' terms and definitions used in ART delivery and evaluation. Having a common terminology is seen as crucial to 'monitoring the availability, efficacy, and safety of assisted reproductive technology' (ibid.: 1521). The application of ARTs in increasingly diverse social, cultural and economic settings makes evermore pressing the need to establish a backdrop of standardised definitions. Without this lingua franca, the mutability of ARTs and their adaptation to different settings will be impeded. Yet, the work of standardisation encompasses far more than mere vocabulary, and extends into training, clinical procedures, appliances, techniques and the drugs used to overcome involuntary childlessness.

In short, the field of ART research, development and delivery is presently characterised by the increasing mobility of personnel, technologies and information. In considering these developments, Knecht and colleagues draw attention to 'reproductive technologies as global form' (Knecht, Beck and Klotz 2012). In so doing, they move beyond local cultures of ARTs and bring into focus an assemblage that is both global and highly influential (Ong and Collier 2005). As this assemblage extends and consolidates, a third phase in the development of ARTs becomes increasingly visible. Speed of diffusion and the proliferation of connection mean that ARTs take on a form that is transnational and distributed with providers and consumers operating outside of state boundaries in the delivery of treatments. Beck, for example, describes the ways in which fertility laboratories in Cyprus are connected by monitors to sites in North America, enabling clinicians to consult and seek advice from more experienced colleagues in the United States. As such, national boundaries appear permeable and incidental to the operation of IVF delivery (Beck 2012). In the same collection, Simpson describes how IVF was established in Sri Lanka in collaboration with international fertility teams. Part of the justification put forward by doctors for establishing services in the country was that access would be widened; those in need of treatment would no longer have to travel abroad and pay overseas rates. Nonetheless, oversight by established UK fertility teams and adherence to international guidelines such as those of the HFEA remained essential for claims made about the comparability and hence the quality of local provision (Simpson 2012). These examples point to an ever-widening repertoire of possibilities for the take-up of knowledge of how to practise ARTs and the markets for equipment and pharmaceuticals on which this diffusion relies. Standard forms of service delivery are thus taken up against diverse legal, demographic and public policy contexts and distinctively local configurations of kinship, gender and well-being.

Bioethical Bricolage and Moral Pioneering

In recent years, public concerns about the ways in which emergent biotechnologies are entering into private lives is currently captured in the field designated as bioethics. As a quasi-secular and liberal discourse on values and meaning in plural societies, bioethics is used as a framework within which to manage complex and sometimes competing claims as to what constitutes progress. In the various contexts that are described in this collection, reproduction emerges as a central preoccupation and, moreover, one linked fundamentally to human flourishing as expressed existentially through ideas of completeness, connection and continuity (van der Geest and Nahar 2013). Not to be able to reproduce when there are strong pressures to do so invites both speculation (why me?) and action (what can we do by way of remedy?). What actions are permissible and encouraged can easily be read off from custom, belief and tradition. For example, although fertility rites and the use of medicines to achieve conception are common in many societies, fostering, adoption, polygamy and other such strategies to acquire children might be resorted to when these fail. Ways of ensuring social reproduction when biological reproduction fails are as old as human society itself. However, where ARTs are concerned, what is forbidden and proscribed is not always clear and is likely to be the subject of debate and negotiation. Evaluating possible courses of action in the face of unwanted infertility invites consideration of multiple reference points of legitimation, engenders novel precedents, and stimulates creative interpretations, all of which are likely to be adduced to bring orthodoxy into line with what Inhorn once referred to as 'immortality desire' (Inhorn 1994a). The result is something akin to the bricolage made famous in Levi Strauss's account of mythological thought and the human imagination (Levi-Strauss 1966). In this view, the human imagination does not operate with a blueprint made up of rules that are straightforwardly observed, but actively and creatively fashions meaning out of diverse and readily available sets of symbolic resources. The resultant forms have the character of being cobbled together in the manner of a contraption that mostly functions adequately rather than a well-built machine that is designed for purpose.

In this regard, we are keen to draw attention to the ways in which the reception of ARTs inspires experimentation and pioneering in the quest for meaning. Infertile couples, their wider families, clerics, physicians and other interested parties engage in the deconstruction and reconstruction of meaning in order to arrive at workable models for how to make sense of misfortune and its remedies. The book thus brings into focus examples of the co-production of moral worlds in which the use of ARTs figures as an acceptable strategy for individuals, families and communities to deal with the distress that comes with unwanted infertility. Through a variety of ethnographic approaches we examine the kaleidoscope of influences that feature in a quest not merely for conception, but for a morally situated conception.

In focusing on the ways in which ARTs are coming within the reach of new constituencies as defined by socio-economic status, ethnicity and geography, we thus seek to move beyond a model that posits a backdrop of standardised delivery in front of which cultural diversity is widely and often problematically acted out. In considering new and emerging arena of engagement with ARTs throughout the world we draw attention to the flow of ideas in both directions. Beliefs and practices designated as 'traditional' or 'cultural' are rendered permeable and labile when individuals are faced with reproductive challenge and the novel solutions on offer. Conversely, medical practices are subject to variation and modification in ways that belie the standard models of clinical and ethical practice when rolled out in culturally and economically diverse contexts.

The Book

This book is divided into three parts, each of which begins with an analytical commentary on the content and cross-cutting themes of the chapters. A novel experiment in the book is to conclude each part with a commentary from those practising in the fields that we have described.

The first part takes up the theme of engagement with ARTs not just as a therapeutic encounter but also as a kind of moral journey. Consistent with the metaphor of journeying is the idea of people moving into new conceptual terrains as 'pioneers' for whom techno-scientific innovation initiates decision making that, in cultural terms, is as risky as it is novel (Rapp 1988). ARTs in the third phase operate in settings in which frameworks of meaning are typically partial, contradictory and emergent. In her overview, Inhorn invites us to consider 'what is most at stake' (to use Kleinman's [2006] terminology) when novel technologies penetrate the diverse local moral worlds of contemporary Islam. The chapters that follow illustrate the nature of the quest for accommodation and legitimation of ARTs within the context of Islam in the broadest sense. However, detailed expositions of the practice of ARTS in religiously plural Lebanon (Clarke), among Pakistani Sunni Muslims in England (Simpson, Blell and Hampshire) and among Shias in Iran and the UK (Tremayne) highlight the variability that underlies any simple claims to an Islamic bioethics or intra-national, let alone inter-national public consensus – a variability that is further underlined by Mahmoud's reflection on his work in the UK as a Muslim practitioner of gynaecology and reproductive medicine. Each of the pieces throws light on the ways in which religious, legal and customary authority is woven into debate, consultation, opinion and decision making to produce workable legitimation of present and future actions regarding family formation. In their effects, ARTs are not simply grafted onto stable forms of family and kinship but are themselves part of the shifting mosaic of relationality in everyday life. Our intention in bringing these chapters together is thus not to essentialise or exceptionalise Islam in relation to the ARTs; indeed, quite the opposite. By juxtaposing pieces on groups of people who all define themselves broadly as Muslims, we see the variation and negotiation that emerges as individuals, couples, families and others encounter and navigate newly emerging and local moral worlds.

In the second part, attention turns to ARTs and infertility in resource-poor areas, with examples drawn from Bangladesh

(Nahar), Botswana (Bochow) and Mali (Hörbst). It opens with an introduction by Trudie Gerrits who, drawing together insights from the other chapters together with reflections from her own recent work in infertility clinics in Ghana, considers what new kinds of questions emerge when ARTs come within reach of new populations, and the reconfigured forms of stratified reproduction and biological citizenship that might result. The chapter by Willem Ombelet then offers a careful reflection on the politics of access to ARTs in the developing world by arguing that it is no longer acceptable that ARTs remain the preserve of those who can afford them. Considering the burden of involuntary childlessness in low-income settings, Ombelet contends that infertility should no longer be seen as an individual medical problem but be recast as a major public health issue and accompanied by a global campaign to alleviate it. His arguments are clearly articulated in terms of reproductive autonomy, social justice and equity as enshrined in World Health Organization strategy regarding family planning. The ethnographic chapters that make up this part each describe ARTs within broader cultural, economic and historical trajectories, and specifically the very contexts in which Ombelet envisages a widening access to ARTs. Papreen Nahar describes how knowledge of infertility treatments in Bangladesh circulate between rural and urban contexts with ARTs featuring as an important imaginary when dealing with infertility – that is, thought about by many but accessed by only a few. The account of ARTs in Gaborone, Botswana, by Astrid Bochow draws on biographies of women of different ages to plot how infertility treatment and ARTs have become established over time. Similarly, Viola Hörbst analyses detailed ART stories of women in Bamako, Mali, to reveal the relationship between the social and financial status of women and their strategies for accessing fertility treatment. In both chapters, the pattern of ART use is initially one of elites accessing treatments outside of the country followed by the development of local provision for such elites and, subsequently, a blending of ART treatments with a range of local provisions. The twist in the tail in Hörbst's account however is the loss of confidence and a shift away from local Malian providers back into the global marketplace of fertility treatment. Both studies highlight the ways in which financial and familial interests shape individual strategies for engagement with ARTs, and in so doing provide important contextual detail regarding the reshaping of reproductive relations in the third phase of ARTs. Finally, the commentary by Thilina Palihawadana and H.R. Seneviratne offers some important insights and reflections into the challenges and dilemmas that private practitioners might confront when establishing ART provision.

The extension of ARTs to new populations and new subgroups (ethnic, socio-economic) within populations raises many questions about interactions between health care professionals and increasingly diverse recipients of these technologies. The third and final part of this book explores the ethics of care from the perspective of ethno-religious communities. Here novel reproductive interventions are taken as the focal point in thinking about professional response to ARTs in diverse cultural and socio-economic settings. The notion of discrete moral worlds that map neatly onto group or community is brought into question in chapters by Sangeeta Chattoo, and Nicky Hudson and Lorraine Culley, in ways that are illuminating for the notion of ARTs in the third phase. Both pieces reflect on the place of ethno-religious communities in the context of UK society in general and health policy in particular, and each sounds a cautionary note when it comes to over-investing in the idea of bounded 'cultures' within which a discrete and ordered morality prevails. Each piece extends the arguments made in the preceding parts, drawing attention to the permeability and scalability of the categories and classifications likely to be in circulation at the interface between health care providers and the communities they serve. Chattoo goes beyond 'minority' groups in order to examine the way that the category 'South Asian' is used by medical professionals in relation to questions of infertility, privacy and autonomy among such groups. Central to her concerns are questions of just what constitutes 'culturally competent care' in the context of NHS delivery, what this tells us about difference, and how in political and ideological terms it is currently being managed. In similar vein, Hudson and Culley, who explore the perceptions of different South Asian 'ethnic communities' (Muslim, Sikh and Hindu) on third-party gamete transactions, show that, while religious and ethnic identities were important in shaping ideas and beliefs, other dimensions such as gender were very important and cut across ethnicity and religion. In her introduction to this part, Alison Shaw invites health professionals to develop 'a sort of *moral imagination*' that is informed by an understanding of the different kinds of values that might be encountered in a culturally and linguistically diverse population, but not to make assumptions based on stereotypes. Crucially, this entails having a critical awareness of the socially constructed nature of one's own values and practices. This call is taken up in the final commentary in the volume by two junior doctors, both of whom incorporated a medical anthropology master's programme into their medical training. Ana Liddie Navarro and Miriam Orcutt describe some of the challenges they face personally when trying to develop this kind of cultural sensitivity and competence as junior doctors in a health system that is relatively inflexible and tightly constrained by time pressures.

In this collection we bring into focus a third phase in the development of ARTs in which access to these extraordinary technologies is beginning to move beyond global elites and is accessed by evermore diverse cultural and socio-economic constituencies using evermore novel strategies. In sketching out the contours of what this development looks like, we highlight some of the ethical and practical complexities that arise in the quest for parenthood in the twenty-first century.

Notes

1. The preferred acronym throughout this piece is ART rather NRT (New Reproductive Technology) as we wish to emphasise the increasing routinisation of assistance in reproductive failure rather than novelty per se.
2. In this case a Canadian woman secured legal permission for a future donation of her eggs to her daughter, who had been rendered infertile as a result of being born with Turner Syndrome (Edwards 2009). Retrieved on 8 August 2011 from http://www.nature.com/news/2007/070702/full/news070702-5.
3. In this case, two gay men have formed a family of five children using their own sperm and the services of egg donors and surrogates. Retrieved on 8 August 2011 from http://www.guardian.co.uk/lifeandstyle/2010/jul/17/gay-fathers-drewitt-barlow. Also see Simpson 2004b for a novel South Asian reading of this case.
4. In the case of Diane Blood, sperm was extracted posthumously from her husband, and using cryopreserved sperm she was able to produce two children over a period of years who were the biogenetic offspring of her dead husband (Simpson 2001b).
5. 'Infertility time bomb' warning given at a 2005 European Fertility Conference by Professor Bill Ledger of the University of Sheffield. Retrieved on 1 June 2011 from http://news.bbc.co.uk/1/hi/health/4112450.stm.

6. WHO, http://www.nice.org.uk/nicemedia/pdf/CG011publicinfoenglish.pdf.
7. The UK's Human Fertilisation and Embryology Authority reports that in 1991, when the authority was established and data collection began, there were 6,146 IVF patients who underwent 6,609 cycles. By 2006 these figures had risen to 18,183 and 22,343 respectively (HFEA 2007). The figure reported by the HFEA for 2010 was 45,246 patients undergoing 57,652 cycles. Retrieved on 12 July 2012 from http://www.hfea.gov.uk/ivf-figures-2006.html.
8. The target of three cycles on demand has mostly become an aspiration, with many trusts being unable to afford any treatments at all (for example, see: 'Rationing Babies: IVF is still a Postcode Lottery'. Retrieved on 30 May 2014 from http://www.independent.co.uk/life-style/health-and-families/health-news/rationing-babies-ivf-is-still-a-postcode-lottery-1682308.html).
9. 'Funding IVF in the UK is Feeble': a BBC News report on comments made by Dr Mark Connelly at ESHRE conference in July 2012. Retrieved on 21 May 2013 from http://www.bbc.co.uk/news/health-18675858.
10. The Pakistani Muslim research was carried out with the aid of a grant from the UK's Economic and Social Research Council (RES-000-23-1488).
11. For example, see newspaper article headlined 'Whites Will be an Ethnic Minority in Britain by the End of the Century' (Browne 2000).

Bob Simpson is a professor of anthropology at the University of Durham. His current research interests focus on bioethics, biomedicine and biotechnologies in developing world contexts. An important geographical focus of his work has been South Asia, where he has explored the encounter between challenging technological developments and local systems of values and beliefs. He has also worked on changing forms of kinship and family formation in the UK, and is the author of *Changing Families: An Ethnographic Approach to Divorce and Separation* (1998).

Kate Hampshire is a reader in Anthropology at Durham University, UK. Kate is a medical anthropologist and works mostly in sub-Saharan Africa. She is currently working on the use of information and communications technologies (ICTs) and therapeutic technologies (particularly medicines) by children and adolescents in Ghana, Malawi and South Africa. A major methodological focus of her work has been to develop innovative ways of working collaboratively with young people, and to facilitate research partnerships with academics and policymakers in the Global South. She has recently co-edited (with Gina Porter and Janet Townsend) a collection, *Children and Young People as Knowledge Producers* (2014).

PART I

(ISLAMIC) ART JOURNEYS AND MORAL PIONEERS

Part I – Introduction

New Reproductive Technologies in Islamic Local Moral Worlds

Marcia C. Inhorn

Moral Pioneers in Local Moral Worlds

In 1988, exactly ten years after the birth of the first test-tube baby, Louise Brown, in England, an American feminist medical anthropologist, Rayna Rapp, published a path-breaking article on 'Moral Pioneers: Women, Men and Fetuses on a Frontier of Reproductive Technology'. While in vitro fertilisation (IVF) was being promoted as a new way of achieving pregnancy among infertile women, amniocentesis was being touted as a way for pregnant women to prevent the birth of disabled children through prenatal diagnosis. By 1988, both of these new reproductive technologies (NRTs) were beginning to be routinised in the US, UK and other Western countries as a way for women to have further 'choices' about their reproduction and motherhood.

However, as Rapp so poignantly articulated in her essay, and later in her award-winning book, *Testing Women, Testing the Fetus: The Social Impact of Amniocentesis in America* (Rapp 1998), women who were being encouraged to adopt amniocentesis to 'control' their pregnancy outcomes (i.e. to abort fetuses with Down syndrome and other genetic defects) were being put in very difficult positions as 'moral pioneers'. As Rapp explained,

> The local meanings of pregnancy, maternity, parental love, and adult gender identity shape the decisions surrounding abortion or the birth of a disabled child. Despite their diversity, retrospective interviews also reveal the common depths of isolation inherent in pursuing the consequences of this new reproductive technology ... Technology here creates a traumatic experience which is so deeply medicalised and privatised that its social shape has yet to be excavated, and a cultural language for its description yet to be found. (Rapp 1988: 111)

Rapp went on to argue that in American culture, 'where science and technology make powerful claims on the transformation of pregnancy and personhood' (ibid.: 114), feminist scholars must take an active role in listening to the discourses of women from a variety of social positions when they are forced to play the role of moral pioneers in their encounters with new reproductive technologies of all kinds. Despite the promotion of these technologies within mainstream Western medicine and the surrounding cultural discourses that valorise 'reproductive choice', Rapp's research was among the first to highlight the difficult moral dilemmas faced by women as they decide whether or not to undertake new reproductive technologies and, once undertaken, how to make sense of the sometimes untoward consequences and outcomes. In short, Rapp introduced the term 'moral pioneers' to capture women's highly fraught moral decision making in the midst of an expanding technological universe of reprogenetics.

Four years later, in 1992, American medical anthropologist Arthur Kleinman expanded upon Rapp's notion of moral pioneering in his seminal article, 'Local Worlds of Suffering: An Interpersonal Focus for Ethnographies of Illness Experience'. In this essay and then in his later two books, *Writing at the Margins: Discourse between Anthropology and Medicine* (Kleinman 1997) and *What Really Matters: Living a Moral Life Amidst Uncertainty and Danger* (Kleinman 2006), Kleinman argued that ethnographers must shed light on what he called 'local moral worlds'. As he explained,

> What precedes, constitutes, expresses, and follows from our actions in interpersonal flows of experience are particular local patterns of recreating *what is most at stake* for us, what we most fear, what we most aspire to, what we are most threatened by, what we most desire to cross over to for safety, and what we jointly take to be the purpose, or the ultimate meaning, of our living and our dying. Nowhere is this moral cast to the flow of experience more recognisably

> influential than in that type of experience of contingent misfortune or routinised misery to which we give the perennially resonant name 'suffering'. (Kleinman 1992: 129)

Through an 'ethnography of experience', Kleinman urged medical anthropologists to pay close attention to moral issues of spiritual pain and social suffering, which may accompany the arrival of new biotechnologies around the globe. Indeed, local moralities are perhaps best exposed when new health technologies confront deeply embedded religious and ethical traditions. Such traditions may embrace new biotechnologies (e.g. blood transfusion, kidney dialysis), but also prohibit others that do not meet with local religious norms (e.g. egg and sperm donation, abortion). For individuals confronting the moral stances and ambiguities of their local religious traditions, they must attempt to make sense of such religious responses, while at the same time invoking their own moral subjectivities to find acceptable solutions to their often dire health needs and concerns.

New Reproductive Technologies in Islamic Local Moral Worlds

Although Rapp's concept of 'moral pioneers' and Kleinman's concept of 'local moral worlds' were developed within a Western setting, the present volume shows the importance of moving these tropes to the Muslim world. In Part I, all three chapters are devoted to Islam and assisted reproduction, showing how practising Muslims must make sense of a dizzying array of reproductive possibilities to overcome their childlessness. These chapters highlight what is at stake for ordinary Muslims as they attempt to make reproductive decisions in a way that is morally satisfying and consistent with local religious norms. In short, these chapters ask: What do Muslim IVF seekers think about making a test-tube baby? And, when faced with the need for donor eggs, sperm, or gestational surrogates to overcome infertility, what do ordinary Muslim men and women actually do? Given the ongoing globalisation of ARTs to the Muslim world, these are all open questions.

Quite importantly, Islamic institutions and individual clerics have provided considerable guidance to Muslim couples as they attempt to overcome their infertility. As early as 1980, the first formal *fatwa*, or authoritative religious decree, on IVF was issued by the Grand Shaykh of Egypt's Al-Azhar University, the world-renowned centre of Islamic learning (Inhorn 2003a, 2012). The Al-Azhar *fatwa* was supportive of IVF, as long as no third parties were used to donate reproductive material (i.e. eggs, sperm, embryos or uteruses, as in gestational surrogacy). IVF clinics thus opened in Egypt, Jordan and Saudi Arabia by 1986, during the very 'first phase' of ART development, per the introduction to this volume. By the 'second phase' of ART globalisation, the Muslim Middle East already boasted one of the strongest ART sectors in the world, a global metric unmatched in virtually any other region outside of the West. Today, there is not a single Middle Eastern country without its own IVF clinic. Furthermore, some of these countries have many clinics – Egypt with more than 50, Iran with more than 70, and Turkey with more than 110. Although other parts of the Muslim world have lagged behind, particularly Muslim countries in sub-Saharan Africa and Central Asia, these technologies are now well ensconced in the most populous Muslim countries, including Indonesia, Malaysia and Pakistan.

Given the rapid technological development and continuous diffusion of new forms of reproductive technology, the time has certainly come to examine the globalisation of ARTs to diverse Islamic contexts. The authors in this part of the volume are among a small group of about a dozen researchers who are engaging in empirical studies of assisted reproduction in the Muslim world (Inhorn and Tremayne 2012).

In general terms, it is fair to say that Islamic religious authorities have condoned IVF, making the technology morally permissible for practising Muslims. Such religious permission has clearly facilitated the aforementioned early development of a 'first phase' IVF industry across the Muslim world. However, it is equally important to point out that not all solutions to childlessness are equally valid from an Islamic standpoint. In particular, third parties of all kinds, whether they be egg, sperm or embryo donors, gestational surrogates or adopted children, are not allowed by Sunni Muslim religious authorities – and Sunnis represent about 90 per cent of the world's Muslims. The Sunni disavowal of third party reproductive assistance draws from diverse moral principles, but revolves around concerns over: purity of lineage and the genealogical confusion introduced by third parties; marriage and the equivalence of third parties with adultery; the possibility of incest among the half-sibling offspring of anonymous donors; and a child's rights to know parentage, with adverse psychological outcomes in the absence of such information.

These are all compelling justifications within the Sunni Islamic local moral world. However, not all Muslims agree with these anti-third-party stances. Indeed, since the new millennium – or what the editors call the 'third phase' of ARTs – there is increasing evidence of discordance and dissent across the Muslim world. Minority religious responses, particularly on the part of Shia Muslims (about 10 per cent of the world's Muslim population), have been a particularly important part of this resistance. For example, in 1999, the Supreme Leader of the Islamic Republic of Iran, Ayatollah Ali al-Hussein al-Khamene'i – the hand-picked successor to Ayatollah Khomeini – issued a *fatwa* allowing donor technologies to be used (Inhorn 2003a; Clarke 2009; Clarke and Inhorn 2011; Inhorn and Tremayne 2012). As a result, since the new millennium, donor gametes and gestational surrogates are now being utilised by infertile couples in IVF clinics in Shia-majority Iran and Lebanon, currently the only two countries in the Muslim world to allow this practice.

In short, Islam, as a global religion, is not monolithic, timeless and unchanging. As noted by James Gelvin in his recent compelling history, *The Modern Middle East*:

> The doctrines and institutions associated with Islam or any other religion are not frozen in time. They exist within history, not outside history. And while there are continuities of religious doctrines and institutions, the meaning those doctrines and institutions hold for society, and the function they play in society, evolve through time. (Gelvin 2005: 292)

In short, if we are to speak of an emerging 'Islamic bioethics' (Brockopp 2003; Brockopp and Eich 2008; Sachedina 2009), then it is important to bear in mind that Muslims do not agree on some set of common global norms or 'best practices'. Islamic local moral worlds are as diverse as the technologies themselves. And when speaking of moral pioneers, it is important to emphasise that not all Muslims make the same moral decisions, nor think alike. Levels of religiosity vary tremendously. Some Muslims are pious, while others are not. Some are scripturally oriented, while others value independent reasoning. Some follow particular clerics, while others consider their primary relationship to be with God. Some know that they are 'rule breaking', but hope for God's mercy and forgiveness. Others simply do not care, having left the religion, or having associated themselves with other traditions such as secular humanism, communism, atheism or 'science'. This great diversity within the world's Muslims cannot be emphasised enough. Muslims do not follow a single path. Their local moral responses are mediated by a wide variety of ever-changing values and social forces.

Islamic Technoscience in Practice

Given the moral complexity of assisted reproduction – which invokes, among many other things, issues of embryo creation and disposition, fetal reduction through abortion, pre-implantation culling of diseased embryos or those of the 'wrong sex', donation of reproductive material between unmarried and anonymous persons, commodification of others' bodies in order to create and carry a child, and so on – the ARTs and Muslims' attitudes towards them provide a compelling nexus for the study of what might be called 'Islamic technoscience in practice'. As noted by anthropologist Mazyar Lotfalian (2004) in his unique volume, *Islam, Technoscientific Identities, and the Culture of Curiosity*, there is a glaring lacuna in the study of science and technology in the Islamic world. According to Lotfalian, there are 'really only two strains of relevant work' – one on the Islamic medieval sciences, and the other on philosophical arguments for civilisational differences between Islamic and Western science and technology (i.e. Samuel P. Huntington's so-called 'clash of civilisations' thesis). This dearth of relevant scholarship clearly applies to the cross-cultural study of ARTs. For example, in the seminal volume on *Third Party Assisted Conception across Cultures: Social, Legal and Ethical Perspectives*, not a single Muslim society is represented among the thirteen country case studies (Blyth and Landau 2004).

This is why the three chapters presented in Part I, all focusing on diverse contexts in the Muslim world, make a major contribution to our understanding of Islamic technoscience in practice. In his chapter '"Islamic Bioethics" in Transnational Perspective', Morgan Clarke takes up the broad task of interrogating the notion of 'Islamic bioethics', a term that is increasingly invoked in scholarship on technoscience and medical practice in Muslim contexts. First, he challenges the idea that there is a discrete body of thought, or a separate academic discipline, which could be called 'Islamic bioethics'. Rather, questions regarding Islam and medicine – usually posed as 'Is X (the medical technique) allowed in Y (Islam)'? – are taken up in the Islamic legal tradition of *fiqh*, or Islamic jurisprudence. However, as emphasised by Clarke, Islamic *fiqh* debates and resulting *fatwas* are *not* the same as an 'Islamic bioethics'.

Instead, Clarke makes a strong argument for the 'local moral': namely, that any notion of Islamic bioethics must be 'reread' in light of local specificities. Clarke has conducted his field research in Lebanon, one of the most religiously diverse countries in the world, or at least in the Muslim world. There, a Shia Muslim majority prides itself on what Clarke calls 'contemporaneity', or 'keeping up with the times'. Part of this contemporaneity is an openness to new scientific and medical innovations, which are discussed, debated and often authorised by local Shia clerics. As a result, Shia Muslims in Lebanon are able to obtain ARTs that are not authorised for use by Lebanese Sunni Muslims. Furthermore, depending upon which cleric is followed, Shia Muslims themselves may differ in their opinions over the uptake of certain technologies, such as egg and sperm donation.

Such local constellations of political, religious and biomedical authority – or what might be called 'the local moral world' of ARTs in Lebanon – should be the focus of scholarly inquiry, according to Clarke. The search for abstract, 'transnational perspectives' on Islamic bioethics, he opines, is a misplaced pursuit. Thus, the title of Clarke's chapter – '"Islamic Bioethics" in Transnational Perspective' – belies the author's actual support of Kleinman's call to arms: namely, that anthropologists must study the 'local moral' over the 'universal bioethical' if they want to understand what is truly at stake in the contemporary world of biomedicine (Kleinman 1997).

In the next chapter, 'Moral Pioneers: Pakistani Muslims and the Take-Up of Assisted Reproductive Technologies in the North of England', authors Simpson, Blell and Hampshire also examine the local moral worlds of the Pakistani Muslim minority population living within a working-class, diasporic British setting. ARTs are widely available in the UK, and receive government support through state subsidisation. However, the 'take-up' of these technologies is not straightforward within the Pakistani Muslim community in northern England. Through field research with both fertile and infertile community members, the authors show that the Pakistani community itself is diverse, with varying levels of education, religiosity, and knowledge about reproduction and ARTs. Nonetheless, 'community' matters. Young Pakistani Muslim couples who experience infertility often face quite invasive and interventionist scrutiny by community members, who may or may not encourage the uptake of ARTs. The authors show that although some 'cosmopolitan' Pakistanis welcome ARTs as a solution to childlessness, others community members, including local imams and some Muslim physicians, may view these technologies with suspicion. Thus, infertile couples are often keen to keep their reproductive problems strictly private, and resort to ARTs in secrecy.

In this chapter, then, we see the emergence of new notions of *couple solidarity* and *companionate marriage* in the face of community pressure to have children; new desires for *reproductive privacy* in the midst of community intervention and surveillance; and new expressions of *ethical personhood* as infertile men and women 'go against the grain' of their communities' social and religious norms. As this chapter shows, infertile British Pakistani Muslim couples are increasingly taking morally pioneering stances by engaging with ARTs that are frowned upon, even condemned, by important members of their local moral worlds. Such resistances to communal authority are incredibly important to any discussion of ARTs and Islam in the new millennium, because such religious resistances seem to be increasing with each new technological development (Inhorn 2012).

In the final chapter, 'Whither Kinship? Assisted Reproductive Technologies and Relatedness in the Islamic Republic of Iran', this theme of resistance is abundantly apparent. For as anthropologist Soraya Tremayne (2009, 2012) has shown in her previous path-breaking work, Iran is leading the way into the brave new world of third-party reproductive assistance, with leading clerics taking morally pioneering decisions in this regard. As a result, Iran is currently the only Muslim country where third-party gamete and embryo donations are widely practised, along with altruistic and commercial gestational surrogacy. Yet, even within this 'permissive' ART environment, certain Islamic rules of kinship are supposed to be maintained. Most importantly, Islamic doctrines are very specific about incest and adultery, dividing men and women into two categories: *mahrams*, who are relatives and are not potential marital or sexual partners, versus *na-mahrams*, who are not relatives, but are potential marital and sexual partners.

What Tremayne is able to show through in-depth field research in Iranian IVF clinics is that infertile Iranian couples are wittingly or unwittingly flouting these kinship rules, sometimes with the tacit aid of doctors. For example, infertile men routinely use their brothers' sperm to impregnate their wives, sometimes without wives' knowledge. Brothers donate sperm to their sisters' infertile husbands, such that the embryos formed are the product of a brother's and sister's gametes. And gestational surrogates are often siblings of the wife or husband, even though commercial gestational surrogacy with third-party surrogates is allowed and available in the country.

Tremayne argues that the introduction of donor technologies and surrogacy in Iran has served to keep reproduction 'all in the family', strengthening kinship bonds. Namely, exchanges of gametes and wombs between family members are seen as consolidating the bonds within the kin group, even if such exchanges are illicit from an Islamic moral perspective, and problematic from a genetic perspective as well. Although the merging of a brother's and sister's gametes in a petri dish might be viewed as 'incest', those infertility patients and physicians who are undertaking these sibling-gamete combinations resist the incest label, arguing that incest has not occurred because no sexual activity has taken place.

In short, within the local moral world of Iranian ARTs, the importance of biological connection is being reinforced, at the same time that Islamic rules of marriage, filiation, descent and incest are being undermined. The future of kinship, Tremayne concludes, is uncertain, because the long-term outcomes of these close-relative donations and bodily exchanges remain to be seen in the lives of the offspring thus produced.

Conclusion

As assisted reproductive technologies become further entrenched in the Muslim world, and as additional forms of biotechnology, including new forms of long-term egg freezing, embryo-produced stem cells, and even human reproductive cloning eventually become available, it will be crucial to interrogate new local moralities, as well as new manifestations of kinship and conjugality that are likely to arise in response to these technological innovations. Thus, as anthropologist of science and technology, David Hess, rightly observes, 'Anthropology brings to these discussions a reminder that the cultural construction of science is a global phenomenon, and that the ongoing dialogue of technoculture often takes its most interesting turns in areas of the world outside the developed West' (Hess 1994: 16).

Marcia C. Inhorn is the William K. Lanman Jr. professor of anthropology and international affairs at Yale University. A specialist on Middle Eastern gender, religion and health issues, Inhorn has conducted research on the social impact of infertility and assisted reproductive technologies in Egypt, Lebanon, the United Arab Emirates and Arab America over the past thirty years. She is the author of five books on the subject, and (co-)editor of nine volumes, including *Medical Anthropology at the Intersections: Histories, Activisms, and Futures* (2012). Inhorn is the founding editor of the *Journal of Middle East Women's Studies* (JMEWS), and co-editor (with Soraya Tremayne) of Berghahn Books' *Fertility, Reproduction and Sexuality* series.

Chapter 1

'Islamic Bioethics' in Transnational Perspective

Morgan Clarke

The globalisation of advanced biomedicine has entailed the globalisation of its attendant ethical controversies. My research has examined, among other things, Islamic debates over assisted conception (Clarke 2009). That was in the context of fieldwork in Lebanon, which has substantial Sunni and Shia Muslim communities. Islamic legal opinion is varied, and frequently strikingly unrestrictive. Some Shia authorities have even permitted such controversial procedures as those involving donor gametes and surrogacy arrangements, most notoriously Ayatollah 'Ali al-Khamene'i, the highly controversial Supreme Leader of the Islamic Republic of Iran.[1] Predominantly Shia, Iran is, besides Lebanon, the only country in the Middle East where donor procedures are available. It has thus proved tempting to take the two together and then draw a broad contrast between 'Sunni' and 'Shia' approaches, paralleling those between, say, 'Islamic' and 'Christian' ones (as I have frequently done, I should say, in my own work; also see Mahmood, this volume).

But to remain with this binary would be to ignore the substantial differences in the ways that religious, medical and state legal authority are related in different contexts, as well as the individual scholarly and political projects such rulings may serve. What are commonly glossed as instances of a free-floating 'Islamic bioethics' thus need to be re-read, I argue here, as distinctive local constellations of such national and transnational relations and projects (see also Clarke 2012a). Only by attending to such local specificities can we truly appreciate the transnational dynamics of the flows of these technologies and the ethical and religio-legal debates that accompany them.

'Islamic Bioethics'

Before turning to my Lebanese cases, let me advance a few brief initial comments about the category 'Islamic bioethics'. There is certainly a considerable appetite, in scholarly and indeed medical circles, for such a thing as an 'Islamic bioethics' (Atighetchi 2007; Brockopp and Eich 2008: 5–7; Shanawani and Khalil 2008). The fascination is, I think, twofold. On the one hand, bioethics and medical ethics have become well-resourced academic disciplines in their own right, to a certain extent parasitic (if I can put it like that) on the very considerable funding, public and private, devoted to biotechnological and biomedical research and practice, and governmental interest in that research and practice. The need for informed policy and regulation of research and medical practice was, according to many commentators, one of the fundamental drivers for the formation of an institutionalised bioethics in its original American forms, the Hastings Centre and the Kennedy Institute (e.g. Jonsen 1998).

At its very crudest, a putative Islamic bioethics would serve here as an answer to a question of the form 'Is X allowed in Y?', where X stands for a controversial medical procedure, such as abortion, and Y for a religious or cultural tradition, such as Islam, which, it is felt, needs to be taken into consideration, more or less seriously, for the proper formulation of policy, governmental or clinical. This is of course a very crude, and inadequate, characterisation of what bioethics now is and can be, as an academic and practical discipline. Nevertheless, this sort of legalistic frame is, I think it is fair to say, the dominant form demanded of a putative 'Islamic bioethics', at least in my own experience, both in academic circles in Britain and elsewhere and within clinical settings in Lebanon. Although not exclusively so, this frame is also the dominant form in academic publications devoted to 'Islamic bioethics' (Rispler-Chaim 1993; Brockopp and Eich 2008: 5–7; Eich 2012).

This emphasis on the legalistic is not coincidental, because such a demand is in fact very readily satisfied by the massively elaborated and vivid tradition of Islamic law, or, more exactly, the Islamic science of *fiqh*, usually glossed as 'jurisprudence'. God's right path through life, the sharia, addresses all aspects of life, and so too then does this human science of *fiqh*, which attempts to diagnose what that right path is (see e.g. Hallaq 2009). This universal address, ranging from ritual precepts, through criminal law, contracts of sale and sexual morality, includes medical issues such as abortion and IVF, or scientific research into stem cells or human cloning, within what is often loosely classified as 'the jurisprudence of medicine' (*fiqh al-tibb*). This is not, however, a separate discipline in its own right, but rather a way of categorising a field of varied elements of the wider Islamic legal discourse, albeit a rapidly burgeoning one. Asking 'Does Islam allow abortion?' is a perfectly legitimate and very common way for a Muslim, as much as an academic researcher, to consult an Islamic scholar. And such questions find a very ready, indeed bewilderingly large, array of answers. When one has an appreciation of just how many Islamic scholars of very different legal schools and traditions there are writing on these topics, one immediately perceives the impossible simplicity in this sort of question: what is this 'Islam' and where is it to be found? And, crucially, who speaks for it? This is not to say of course that to ask such questions is merely naive: answers to them of some sort are no doubt needed if good policy is to be made.

Now it is important to note that Islamic concerns over such issues are not merely confined to legalistic assent or denial of the permissibility of carrying out such procedures: that would hardly constitute an ethics of medical practice, even if in many clinical contexts it is taken as sufficient for one, and there is much Islamic scholarship (as well as practical initiatives such as the Muslim doctor's oath)[2] that takes a rounder view of what is required here (Sachedina 2009; Tappan 2012). Beyond the medical domain, it would equally be a mistake to reduce the ethical dimensions of Islam generally to legalistic forms. An important body of recent anthropological scholarship, inspired by Foucault's later writings, has in fact sought to focus attention away from 'jurisprudence' per se and onto individual and institutionalised projects for the formation of virtuous selves (see Clarke 2012b for a recent survey, and Laidlaw 2002 for references to the relevant portions of Foucault's work). Nevertheless, *fiqh* (jurisprudence) is of course a very important tool in that regard, and it is true to say, I think, that it is the predominant form of Islamic ethical discourse, within and without medical and scientific research concerns.

The second source of fascination for 'Islamic bioethics', away from this concrete demand for legalistic pronouncements readily satisfied in Islamic law, springs from the perceived tension within the European and Atlantic traditions between religion and secular modernity, with which 'science' and scientific rationalism are commonly perceived to be inextricably tied. Religion and science are nominally opposed. The frequently enthusiastic and open attitude of many (perhaps even most) Islamic scholars to medical and scientific innovation – which I will present some instances of here – thus never fails, in my experience, to garner academic interest as in some sense surprising: 'So they allow IVF – and some allow cloning?!' This dialectic is not of course confined to Western academic perception. 'Modernity', or the lack of it, has been the pre-eminent focus of social and political concern outside of the West, under colonial rule and now within the post-colony. And this nominal tension between religion and modernity is absolutely central to the dynamics of the contemporary Islamic tradition, which is determined not to be consigned to the dustbin of history as 'backward' and incompatible with scientific modernity as Christianity has been in Europe, according to these Islamic perspectives at least (Clarke 2009: 94). 'Bioethics' is thus in this sense a deeply political issue, while not being directly challenging to the autocratic and frequently repressive regimes of the Middle East, giving room for manoeuvre and debate.

Keeping Up with the Times in Lebanon

Certainly in my own research in Lebanon, to which I now turn, I found that medical ethics, as interpreted through religious traditions, formed an important arena for contests over 'modernity'. In the Lebanese context, religious identity is certainly a topic of key, if not exclusive concern. In something of a hangover from Lebanon's Ottoman past, consolidated under French Mandate rule and then independence, Lebanon's eighteen official religious communities – five Muslim, twelve Christian and one Jewish – enjoy considerable formal autonomies and prerogatives, including, for example, religious tribunals with more or less exclusive jurisdiction over personal status law (Clarke 2012b). Further, under prevailing power-sharing agreements, political office and patronage are distributed on sectarian lines, despite numerous challenges to this privileging of religious identity that lies, so its critics argue, at the root of Lebanon's recent, tragic sectarian conflicts. Nevertheless, it should be noted, these religiously construed privileges are subject to the overarching framework of the Lebanese republic: Lebanese politics cannot be reduced to inter-sect relations, even if some of its most powerful actors – I am thinking especially of the Shia Hezbollah, which I will be discussing further – are explicitly 'religious' organisations.

Religious authorities thus have a relatively high public profile. And one pole around which debate as to their relative merits turns is the extent to which they can be perceived as more or less 'contemporary' (*mu'asir*) and able to 'keep up with the times': perceived contemporaneity can be an important asset. Assisted reproduction, I found in fieldwork in 2003/4, is one such area. Here, the most frequently drawn comparison in clinical circles is between the 'Christian', paradigmatically Catholic position – under which any medical intervention in human reproduction is, broadly speaking, forbidden – and the 'Islamic' one, which allows such intervention as contraception and IVF, albeit within variously defined limits. One pious Shia Muslim medical practitioner, for instance, told me that she had seen 'in the round tables that the Christians are behind here'. This is as much a source of internal as external critique: 'Let the Church accept contraceptive pills and then we'll talk about IVF', as a Christian doctor put it to me. Between the Islamic communities, a similar sub-rivalry then plays out, where the Shia, long marginalised within Lebanese society and denigrated for their perceived 'backwardness' (*takhalluf*), claim a greater rationality and flexibility to their school's brand of Islamic law, due to the nominal relative freedom of their religious specialists to exercise their own independent reasoning (*ijtihad*) in interpreting scripture and the greater weight placed on human reason (*'aql*) as a legitimate source for generating religious law. Lebanon's own late (Shia) Ayatollah Muhammad Husayn Fadlallah (d. 2010), for instance, who made 'open-mindedness' and contemporaneity a pillar of his distinctive appeal, notoriously came out in favour of allowing research into human cloning when the issue became a hot topic in the global media (Clarke 2009: 66, 85n21).

So too did the Supreme Leader of the Islamic Republic of Iran, Ayatollah 'Ali Khamene'i, then widely followed as a religious authority among Lebanese Shia due to the popularity of the Iranian-backed Hezbollah, despite his relatively low scholarly standing in clerical circles (Clarke and Inhorn 2011).[3] At the time of my research in 2003/4 and later in 2007/8, Hezbollah held tremendous prestige and power in Lebanon due to their monopoly over armed resistance to Israel, whose occupation of South Lebanon they claim to have defeated, and to their extensive networks of social provision. Hezbollah acknowledges Khamene'i as their *marja'*, or 'source' of authoritative religious opinion and as the *wali faqih*, or ruling cleric, even if there is no realistic prospect of multi-confessional Lebanon itself becoming an Islamic state. Khamene'i's opinion on assisted reproduction in particular has become notorious: like almost all other Islamic authorities, Sunni as well as Shia, he allows artificial insemination and IVF per se, but, more unusually, he also allows the use of donor eggs and surrogacy arrangements and, almost uniquely and scandalously by the standards of wider society, he allows the use of donor sperm, tantamount to adultery (*zina*) in most eyes and a mighty sin (he argues, among other things, that a medical procedure is in no way equivalent to the sexual act; see Clarke 2007).

The Political Dimension

The comparative 'openness' and 'contemporaneity', in bioethical matters at least, of Shia legal debate was an important theme that emerged from my research. What I want to stress again here is its political currency: such open and contemporary opinions are material to contests over the image and influence of religious authorities, who are often highly politicised figures in this Shia Lebanese context. And while Khamene'i's permission of donor procedures is an important ruling for infertile Shia seeking paths to fertility in what is a highly pro-natal society, this is, it has to be admitted, a relatively marginal domain. There are more obvious ways in which Hezbollah affiliates claim contemporaneity, and hence political effectiveness, through ready engagement with and appropriation of medical and scientific advance.

At the most basic level, the Hezbollah-linked Martyrs' Association runs a major hospital, Al-Rassoul al-'Azam, in Beirut's southern suburbs, where women are required to wear hijab (modest apparel, 'the veil'), and from which at election times patients and staff are reportedly ferried to and from polling stations (Deeb 2006: 115; Harik 2006: 275). Elsewhere in the public sphere, one of the key battlegrounds for Shia reformists has been over the symbolically crucial arena of Ashura, the annual commemoration of the martyrdom of Imam Husayn at Karbala, Iraq, in 680 AD, emblematic of the Shia faith and a core resource for the mobilisation of Shia identity. Nominally 'traditional' practices of self-mortification during the commemorations, such as flagellation and the cutting of the head with razors or swords, have long been the target of reformists (Deeb 2006: 129–64). Ayatollah Khamene'i came out with an explicit authoritative statement of opinion (*fatwa* [pl. fatawa]) condemning them, and further encouraged the substitution of this blood-letting with blood donation, which has become a highly popular alternative in Lebanon (Shaery-Eisenlohr 2008: 135–36, 247n27).

In a sermon given during Ashura in 2008 (when I had returned to Lebanon for further fieldwork on another project), broadcast on Hezbollah's global satellite television station 'al-Manar', Sayyid Hasan Nasrallah, secretary general of Hezbollah, a powerful orator and then a revered figure for many in Lebanon and beyond for his leadership of 'the resistance', gave a distinctively contemporary twist to the established theology of death and martyrdom central to the commemorations, in describing the 'the agonies of death' (*sakarat al-mawt*) endured when, at the fatal moment the angel of death comes and pulls out (*tanza'*) the soul from the body, 'from all [its] cells and nerves', likening it to 'When you go to the dentist to have a tooth removed and the dentist takes out the nerve. How much you suffer from the top of your body to the very bottom from this one little nerve! So how do you think it is when the soul has to be pulled out from every cell?' The biomedical imagery was striking, a harnessing of scientific to religious imagery in the pursuit of political rhetoric that was in this instance, according to my clerical sources, all Nasrallah's own.

To take a more homely example from the same year, in a phone-in programme on the sharia, Hezbollah's radio station 'al-Nur' (91.9 FM), featuring Shaykh Muhammad Tawfiq al-Muqdad, Ayatollah Khamenei's jurisprudential representative in Lebanon, Shaykh Muqdad discussed the topic of the *'awra*, the private parts of the body that should never be revealed; not even other women should see a woman's *'awra* for instance. 'What about the doctor?' asked the presenter (obviously an important issue as regards fertility treatment, for instance). 'Yes,' said the Shaykh, 'a female doctor can look at the *'awra* of the woman. And of course, they are common: but it is not allowed to go to a male doctor'. While in an earlier age for a woman to submit to such an examination by a man would have been a scandalous breach of Islamic morality, the overwhelming prestige of modern medical science has led many to cast such scruples aside. The more recent advent of female education and labour, vital to 'Islamic modernists' for the putative creation of a properly gendered public sphere, has led to the widespread availability of female doctors at the service of Muslim women. But sexist preconceptions of the relative competence of male and female doctors endure, as was clear from the series of callers that rang repeatedly asking permission for their wives to visit male doctors instead, much to Shaykh Muqdad's disgust: 'This talk which I am hearing, that "By God, women doctors don't have skill and proficiency in their profession like men" – this is superstition, it's heresy [*hartaqa*], with no basis in truth. It's not acceptable'.[4]

Shia Islamic Religious Authority

So here, a radical and contemporary vision of Islamic law, to which medicine and science are crucial, is deemed essential to revolutionary progress and is vigorously disseminated via Hezbollah's powerful media outlets, part of a broader project to create what anthropologist Lara Deeb (2006) calls an 'enchanted modern' in Beirut's predominantly Shia southern suburbs. But what I want to probe in the second half of this chapter is precisely whether 'modernity' is really an apposite characterisation of the structures of religious authority in play here. One has to tread carefully; 'modernity' is as much an evaluative as a descriptive term, and my analytical aim should not be misread as an attempt to denigrate, or to praise, the objects of my analysis. Some scholars have tried to avoid this problem by talking of 'alternative modernities' (Gaonkar 2001) – alternative, that is, to the hegemonic Western brand, which is in itself of course differentiated. I am not wholly convinced that gives quite the analytical purchase that one needs here. And the Islamic scholars in whom I am interested are in fact themselves rather shy of ascribing 'modernity' (in Arabic, *hadatha* perhaps) to their project, so easily conflated with Westernisation. I would in fact prefer to follow local rhetoric in calling this orientation one of 'contemporaneity'; that is, 'keeping up with the times' (*muwakibat al-'asr*) rather than the radical break with tradition that modernity implies.

Let me start by focusing more closely on the kinds of statements that are often, somewhat loosely, classified as examples of

'Islamic medical ethics' or 'Islamic bioethics'. Again, there is no such separate discipline. Questions as to the permissibility of new techniques such as IVF fall within the wider purview of *fiqh*, or 'jurisprudence', which is a scholarly pursuit. Any scholar with the appropriate qualifications can engage with the issues and scripture to evolve an opinion on, for example, whether or not IVF with donor sperm is permissible. Those qualifications are, in the Shia case, admittedly exacting. After years of study, one has to be deemed capable by one's scholarly peers of exercising *ijtihad* (independent reasoning) in interpreting scripture in its totality. Of these *mujtahids*, a limited number gain popular acclaim as 'sources' (*maraji'*) of authoritative sharia opinion. Such figures are thus not, within their field, specialists, as a fully developed Weberian vision of rationalised authority might require – as 'bioethicists', for example – their orientation towards the sharia and grasp of it are comprehensive. Their pronouncements on such matters arise, just as the answers of the more junior Shaykh Muqdad, in response to queries of all sorts from their lay followers, nowadays in fact mostly received through electronic media, as emails to their websites, and mediated through their staff (Clarke 2010). These are particular responses to particular questions and cases, often elliptical, sometimes frustratingly so. Responses are never programmatic, comprehensive presentations of 'policy'.

A case in point is Khamene'i's notorious *fatwa* on donor insemination, reproduced in an authoritative collection widely available in Arabic in Beirut, and to be found on some doctors' shelves ready to answer patients' worried queries. Asked by an anonymous petitioner, 'Is it allowed to fertilise the wife of an infertile man with the sperm of a stranger [*rajul ajnabi*, i.e. a man other than her husband], by placing the sperm in her womb?' Khamene'i replies:

> There is no legal obstacle [*la mani' shar'an*] to the fertilisation of the woman with the sperm of a stranger in itself, but forbidden preliminary actions such as looking and touching must be avoided. And in any case, if a child is born in this way, it is not related to the husband, but to the producer of the sperm and to the woman, who is [here] the owner of the egg and the womb. (Khamene'i 2006: part 2: 70; and see Clarke 2007 and 2009: 117–25)

This is terse, to say the least – the expert spares the layperson the details of the debate, of which there are, one should say, a very great many. Some commentary is surely required: prohibited looking and touching refers to the impermissibility of an unrelated male seeing or manipulating the woman's private parts, problematic in the case of such a medical procedure, as we have already seen. Also, the child will be related to the sperm donor rather than the woman's husband, which raises a whole set of other legal, religious and social considerations (Clarke 2009: 121–22). We will surely struggle, then, to perceive such a statement as an instance of 'Islamic bioethics', if by that we mean a separate discipline instituted to generate an intellectual framework ultimately for the generation of policy recommendations.

Take another such petition sent in 2007 to the website (www.bayynat.org) of Ayatollah Fadlallah, eminently 'contemporary' as we have already noted. The correspondent talks of looking for a 'legal loophole' or 'way out' (*manfadh shar'i*) of his dilemma. After divorcing an earlier wife, he suffered from the atrophy of one of his testicles and became totally infertile. He travelled abroad and married another woman, telling his new wife that he could no longer have children, which she accepted. But then they came to Lebanon and she found the social stigma of not being able to have children unbearable. As Fadlallah did not, unlike Khamene'i, allow the use of donor sperm, the response of his offices was that: 'The problem will not be solved except by her divorce from you, and her marriage to someone else, the placing of the sperm of that person in her womb by insemination, then her divorce from him, waiting until the delivery of the pregnancy and then remarrying you'. (And again the child would in fact be considered that of the second husband, the provider of the sperm.)[5]

These sorts of 'ruses', a casuistry addressing individual dilemmas, are paralleled in the possibilities extended by the Islamic permission of polygamy: a man could marry an egg donor or surrogate to remove any suspicion of adultery; under Shia precepts that could even be a temporary marriage, of say 24 hours for an egg donation, for instance (Clarke 2009: 119; Clarke and Inhorn 2011: 422–23). This is individually liberating, but again we can hardly see such responses to followers in ethical need as policy recommendations intended to shape the regulation of medical practice as in British or American bioethical committees. Nevertheless, Fadlallah was famously ready to engage with medical audiences and sought medical advice before forming his opinions. One doctor told me in 2004: 'Fadlallah is a friend, he calls and asks questions. Once he rang about the woman's orgasm. A woman, who had lost her husband, and didn't want to commit adultery, had asked if masturbation negates the Ramadan fast, like for men. That is, is it ritually polluting – that is the case for menstruation, but what about vaginal sexual secretion? I told him no, it's like sweating, a transudate, it has no gamete'. And Fadlallah's subsequent permission of female masturbation was in fact one of his most notorious opinions (Clarke 2009: 147n35).

Regulation of ART in Lebanon and the Wider Region

But, even if this is not regulation, it has an effect on it, albeit a negative one, in the sense of impeding it (although for a libertarian, that would of course be a positive outcome). A proposed law to regulate fertility treatment in Lebanon was drafted by leading medical figures, but in order to get it through parliament, due to Lebanon's confessionalised power-sharing agreement it would have to have been scrutinised by the different religious constituencies – '18 sub-committees' as the doctor in charge put it; that is, one for each of Lebanon's official religious communities – and, as we have seen, opinion is split even within the Shia community, let alone between them and the Catholics. Assisted reproduction is (or was when I last checked) thus essentially unregulated in formal terms – and doctors, both Muslim and Christian, by and large follow the globalised medical ethical precepts of the Western countries where they specialised in these techniques, and leave individual religio-ethical decisions to their patients, who, where religiously committed (which by no means all Lebanese are) turn for guidance to people like Ayatollah Fadlallah, in the case of Shia Muslims, or their parish priest in the case of Christians (Clarke 2009: 163–66).

Doctors in Lebanon are thus free to offer procedures that are regarded as controversial in much of the rest of the region, paradigmatically those involving donor gametes, sperm and eggs. The demand for donor sperm has lessened since the advent of ICSI (intracytoplasmic sperm injection), where just a single sperm is required to fertilise an egg. Donor insemination was in any case a deeply unattractive option for most: just as callers to Shaykh Muqdad's radio show were worried by his insistence on their wives going to a female doctor, so too do many have their doubts about Ayatollah Khamenei's permission of donor insemination, and very few infertile Shia men have in fact been keen to take it up. (And it is worth noting that despite the attention I am paying to these authorities, their influence is very far from overwhelming.) But donor eggs, also allowed by Khamene'i among other Shia authorities, are an important resource for infertile women, and one favoured by many doctors in Lebanon – Muslim and Christian. Several clinics offer this service, and there is considerable demand for it, although, it should be said, it remains controversial and not the preferred choice (Inhorn 2006a; Clarke and Inhorn 2011).

Lebanon has thus also become an attractive destination for so-called 'donor tourists' within the wider region, where, within the context of a booming assisted reproduction sector, such procedures are generally banned, nominally in accord with the precepts of the predominant Sunni school (Inhorn 2011). The majority of Sunni scholars do not allow procedures involving parties other than a husband and one wife, and this majority opinion has translated into effective regulation prohibiting them. The only other country in the region where one can access donor eggs is predominantly Shia Iran. It has thus proved tempting to draw a broad contrast between 'restrictive' Sunni and more 'liberal' Shia positions. While that contrast has some salience in very broad terms in the field of religious discourse, and may have a certain crude effectiveness in terms of practical clinical considerations, it must be heavily qualified. Besides its unfortunate sectarian overtones, it conceals something extremely important: the varied terrain of religious and state authority.

For one thing, the reasons why it is possible to undertake a donor egg procedure in Lebanon or Iran are very different. Lebanon has no regulation to prevent the practice because of a legislature whose politics frequently turn on religious identity, a diversity of religious traditions accompanied by a rhetoric of mutual respect, and the lack of agreement between and even within those traditions concerning the ethics of assisted reproduction: strongly independent practitioners within an almost entirely private medical sector are free to take their own line, and frequently leave ethical decisions to their patients; those Shia legal opinions that permit egg donation are situated within that particular context. Iran, on the other hand (as I understand it, and I am not an expert), has not only state-sponsored regulation but also state-supported fertility clinics and research facilities, which are situated within an important nationalist political agenda: namely, to make Iran a leading site of biomedical research, as is the case regarding human embryonic stem cells, with the explicit blessing of the Supreme Leader, Ayatollah Khamene'i (Saniei 2012). Donor embryo and egg treatments have been permitted in Iranian state law following clerical consultation in committee, noteworthy in itself, given my preceding discussion of personalised religious authority. The use of donor sperm has, however, not been allowed, despite Khamene'i's permission (Abbasi-Shavazi et al. 2008; Tremayne 2009; Garmaroudi 2012). So it is the machinery of the centralised bureaucratic state, here a nominally 'Islamic' state, that counts. In neither case, Lebanon or Iran, should we over-read the formal importance of Khamene'i's or others' opinions.

Similarly, with regard to the putative contrast with the 'Sunni' view, one can in fact find any and every permutation of opinion amongst the innumerable multiplicity of voices within 'Sunni Islam', which includes more than a billion Muslims and a very considerable proportion of the worldwide web's domains. In 2009, I was discussing my research with a Lebanese Sunni sharia court judge, a distinguished and respected scholar, and to my surprise he told me that he himself found the use of donor sperm unexceptionable – a view diametrically opposed to the public 'consensus'. He is not alone in standing apart: the eminent al-Azhar University in Cairo seemingly bubbles with opinions allowing surrogacy, for instance; and one can cite distinguished authorities who see no problem with exploiting Islam's permission of polygamy to allow a man to use the eggs of one wife to fertilise the womb of another (Clarke 2009: 107, 109–10n12).

This vast domain of opinion and debate notwithstanding, an 'official' opinion has nevertheless emerged, official enough to be reflected in the uniform ban, parliamentary or clinical, on the practice of third-party donor procedures and surrogacy arrangements throughout the Sunni-majority Middle East (Inhorn, Patrizio and Serour 2010). Again, it is the ways in which religious and political authority are organised that is in fact salient here. Emblematic of the Ottoman Empire, state muftis (issuers of *fatawa*) are, post-independence, a common feature in these countries. Such state-sponsored muftis are frequently perceived to have been suborned by their political masters. But in the case of medical regulation at least, a close relation between practitioners, the religious establishment and the state as in Egypt, for instance, has been more effective at establishing and policing such standards than the much more differentiated and informal situation in Lebanon (ibid.).

More significant still is the emergence of specialised committees established specifically to overcome what may be perceived as a dangerously confused multiplicity of opinion through the issuing of collectively agreed *fatwa*s: most influential have been those instituted by the Muslim World League in Mecca and the

Organization of the Islamic Conference in Jeddah. The output of these committees is impersonal, and more bureaucratic in form than the responses cited above: a numbered series of points and prescriptions addressing potential dilemmas rather than actually existing individual ones (cf. Eich 2012). This looks much more like an attempt at regulation, albeit in this case from without the state and certainly more like the production of a bioethics committee, although these committees cover the whole range of Sharia topics.

These committee publications, if still termed *fatwa*, nominally emerge from a very different institutional base than those of the Shia *maraji'* we have considered here – and more modern perhaps, in Weberian terms, even if less 'contemporary' in the terms of public perception in Lebanon. One might note, at this point, that regulation by committee would seem almost inevitably to tend towards conservativism. The more conservative opinion tends to emerge as the compromise, as can be seen, for instance, from the changing position of the Muslim World League's council as regards the transfer of gametes within polygynous marriages: initially allowed on the word of one leading scholar, it was later forbidden after the outcry of others (Clarke 2009: 107). Looking more widely, Roman Catholic opinion has become the benchmark for religious ethical debate across the religious traditions by virtue of its tight organisation and standardisation. It also, not coincidentally, most often holds the most conservative position.

Most recently, it should be noted, bioethical committees proper have emerged in the region, as in the national bioethics committees of Tunisia, Egypt and Saudi Arabia. These unite medical, scientific and civil specialists, while paying due deference to the Islamic legal tradition (Eich 2012).

Conclusion

So, while there is a considerable scholarly appetite for an 'Islamic bioethics' with which to do transnational comparative work, and a ready fund of material to satisfy that appetite, some caution is required. The very possibility of the existence of a discipline of 'bioethics', as I take it, entails the distinctive social and political organisation of late modernity: a specialised, expert academic venture, dependent on governmental and biotechnological-industrial funding, evolving policy to be enacted by centralised government or biomedical authority. It entails, that is, certain constellations of power and authority. Now it is not that analogous constellations have not been forged, or attempted to be forged, in contexts outside of the hegemonic West. Modernisation and centralised bureaucratic state organisation are rampant across the world, and certainly within the Middle East, which I am focusing on here. The scientific and medical establishments within the region are frequently highly developed and extremely powerful, as in Iran, for instance. And, as I have just noted, institutions of religious authority can be, and have been, reformed and reinserted into new institutions for the production of ethical output.

If 'Islamic bioethics' are to be a focus of scholarly investigation, then its proper object would be these emerging constellations of relations between political, religious and biomedical authority, in self-ascribed 'Islamic' settings. 'Islamic bioethics', exactly as 'Jewish bioethics', 'Christian bioethics' or 'Buddhist bioethics', would thus be constituted by those distinctive patterns of social relations, more than by any 'religious' or scriptural content (see also Simpson 2004c, 2009). What I was so taken by in Lebanon was not, then, according to this reading, 'Islamic bioethics', but rather the rich and fascinating domain of Islamic legal debate around new medical and scientific issues, which certainly deserves the utmost research and interest, and the ways in which it was related to individual and clinical ethical practice, according to different – more classical, if you like – patterns of authority.

In saying that what I found in Lebanon was not 'Islamic bioethics', I do not mean to imply a lack, as is so commonly alleged, of so-called Orientalist scholarship. That is, in this case, a lack of 'bioethics', for which read 'modernity'. The Islamic legal tradition's long independence, more or less, from state control, its openness, and its closeness and receptivity to everyday concerns, made it, according to some scholars, a bottom-up legal and social project that might be favourably compared to the top-down impositions of the modern nation-state. This independent tradition was a hard-fought-for triumph rather than a failure of development, according to leading academic scholar of Islamic law Wael Hallaq (2009) at least. That independence is, however, contested within the contemporary tradition itself. I should note that the Shia clerical community on which I have focused here is split between those who would preserve the independence of the scholars of the sharia, and those who would subordinate that independence to the demands of the centralised state. And despite the uses to which I have put his work here, Ayatollah Khamene'i is, I should say, in fact the pre-eminent representative of the latter (Khalaji 2006: 22–24, 27–31).

In debating 'Islamic bioethics' then, we are not investigating the ways in which faith can relate to reason. Rather, we are exploring the social relations and institutions through and in which different forms of authority are accumulated and distributed. Only by close attention to distinctive local constellations of such relations and institutions can we hope to understand the dynamics of the transnational practice of reproductive medicine.

Acknowledgements

Many thanks are due to all those who helped me in my researches in Lebanon. The research and writing of this article were funded by an ESRC doctoral studentship at Oxford, a British Academy postdoctoral fellowship at Cambridge and a Simon fellowship at Manchester. Fieldwork was carried out in Lebanon in 2003/4 and 2007/8. Circumstances in Lebanon and the wider region have since changed in ways that would be hard to reflect in detail here.

Notes

1. At the time of writing, Khamene'i's future, and that of the Supreme Leadership, was uncertain following the mass protests against his rule in Iran subsequent to the 2009 presidential elections and their repression.
2. http://www.islamset.com/ethics/code/oath.html, retrieved 5 January 2012.
3. It remains to be seen what impact, if any, his association with the repression of Iran's opposition movement and Hezbollah's implication in the conflict in Syria have in this regard.
4. For more on these two examples, see Clarke 2012a.
5. The example is number 70,324 in the website archive. For a fuller exposition and discussion, see Clarke 2012a.

Morgan Clarke is an associate professor in Social Anthropology at Oxford University. He is an anthropologist with a research focus on the Arabic-speaking Middle East. He has a particular interest in contemporary Islam, especially Islamic law and its relationship to positive law, secular ethics and the civil state.

Chapter 2

Moral Pioneers

Pakistani Muslims and the Take-up of Assisted Reproductive Technologies in the North of England

Bob Simpson, Mwenza Blell and Kate Hampshire

> Dialogism argues that all meaning is relative in the sense that it comes about only as a result of the relation between two bodies occupying simultaneous but different space, where bodies may be thought of as ranging from the immediacy of our physical bodies, to political bodies and to bodies of ideas in general (ideologies).
>
> – Michael Holquist, *Dialogism: Bakhtin and His World*

Moral Pioneering and ARTs

What are the ethical issues faced by British Pakistani Muslims when they contemplate the use of ARTs in the face of difficulties conceiving a child? Are there particular areas of friction and sensitivity that might inhibit access to otherwise widely available treatment? These were the key questions we set out to answer as we embarked on research into the use of ARTs by women and men from this community. At the outset, our question was one that Morgan Clarke has characterised elsewhere in this volume as follows: 'Is X allowed in Y?' where X stands for a controversial medical procedure such as abortion, and Y for a religious or cultural tradition, such as 'Islam', which, it is felt, needs to be taken into consideration, more or less seriously, for the proper formulation of policy, governmental or clinical (Clarke, this volume). In the research we expand on here, 'Y' is a community of Pakistani Muslims living in an industrial town in the north-east of England who share a country of origin and profess the same religion. 'X' is a novel and potentially ethically challenging suite of medical interventions (ARTs) into a condition of common concern (infertility). Along with Clarke, we have found this widely used formulation, and the resulting invocation of a singular 'Islamic bioethics', to be a crude one. The community we encountered did indeed have markers of ethnicity and shared attributes of culture, but the level of engagement and shared intimacy that the topic of infertility generated resulted in far greater texture than is revealed by the 'Is X allowed in Y' question (also see Hampshire, Blell and Simpson 2012a, 2012b). Indeed, as we go on to demonstrate here, the content of our interviews and interactions caused us to question ideas of the clearly bounded and homogenous communities that are often implicit in the methodologies used to study ethnic minorities in plural societies (cf. Shaw and Chattoo, this volume). In our interviews we were struck by the way the responses we received were strongly influenced both by generational, educational, familial and occupational factors, and by the particularities of individuals' lives.

Furthermore, reflection on reproductive narratives suggests other limitations to the 'Is X allowed in Y' question. The ethical framing of ARTs does not happen in a single moment, nor does it suggest a linear trajectory that results in simple acceptance or rejection. On the contrary, the engagement with ARTs for this community, as for any other, is kaleidoscopic in the sense that patterns of ideas and attitudes change according to what people think, what they think others think, what they think others think about what they think and so forth. This approach takes us far from a clear set of prescriptions for action and into the fluid and contingent nature of decision making when suffering is situated in moral worlds. As Inhorn pointed out at the beginning of this part, these moral worlds are not simply 'local' in the sense that Kleinman (1992 and 1997) proposed. Moreover, they are shot through with the influences that come from overarching structures of health care, education and welfare, and through which minority groups become, to greater or lesser degrees, woven into the fabric of Western states and economies.

To draw attention to these exchanges as they arise in the context of interviews and discussions opens up novel ways of bringing together anthropology, ethics and rhetoric. Rather than considering 'attitudes' and 'opinions' as fully formed and final 'monologic utterances' (Bakhtin 1981: 270), we draw attention to reflection, deliberation, reasoning and argumentation, and the role that a variety of reference groups and audiences play as couples describe their predicaments. This is not the abstract reasoning found among Shia Muslim clerics (*ijtihad*) (Clarke 2009), but the more prosaic and day-to-day efforts to integrate desires and expectations that are not always consistent with one another. In this view, social life, and by extension ethical life, are ongoing projects in which individuals and groups attempt to persuade one another of the self-evidence, correctness, truth, authenticity and wisdom of one way of living in the world over another. As Carrithers puts it: 'in any moment of interaction, some act to persuade, others are the targets of persuasion; some work, others are worked upon' (Carrithers 2005: 580). In discussions about infertility, and whether certain courses of action were morally acceptable or not, it was noticeable how couples readily invoked absent others and imaginary audiences for their actions, and even for their thoughts. This dynamic and processual view of social and ethical life draws into question the view of culture as a repertoire of codes and rules to be followed, and focuses instead on the day-to-day work of creating the appearance of stable and structured systems that people can inhabit with a reasonable degree of order and predictability. The phenomenologist Alfred Schütz characterised those who are directly engaged in this process as consociates, or those with whom an individual is in ongoing face-to-face relations (Schütz [1932] 1967). Of more relevance for the argument developed here, however, Schütz identifies an important role for those who lie beyond immediate experience. These are the audiences and publics who are outside the immediate social world (contemporaries), those who went before (predecessors) and those who it is imagined will come after (successors), all of whom play their part in enabling people to arrive at ethical positions that are felt to be consistent with prevailing social and cultural values.

In Pakistani Muslim accounts of ARTs, we might thus identify a range of audiences that couples feel inclined or possibly obliged to address in their accounts. Bakhtin's dialogism is useful in capturing the dynamic at work; utterances are characterised by their 'addressivity' – that is, they are directed towards specific audiences. They also are marked by their 'answerability', anticipating certain answers and responses in the move towards a sense of ethical responsibility for actions taken or about to be taken. Following Schütz we can readily see such dialogues taking place with consociates: family and kinship networks, the local community and wider networks in the UK and overseas accessed directly or with the help of new and powerful information and communication technologies. However, there are also wider referents beyond the contexts of face-to-face communication. Schütz's contemporaries are evident in references to the wider Pakistani diaspora and communities 'back home'. We might also include here new contemporaries such as the medical profession and a variety of educators whose influence is evident in people's cogitations.

Predecessors appear regularly in references to parents and grandparents here and abroad. Successors occupy a particularly powerful place in this account, for they are the wished for progeny that will continue the lineage, uphold the religion and, as future moral persons, honour their parents and their predecessors. Thinking about the role of audiences in this way is helpful in illuminating the complex operations that underpin the making of moral justification and consensus around the use of assisted reproductive technology to address childlessness within this and other communities. However, viewed in this way there is a strong presumption of convergence. In the face of contention and contradiction, we can identify a strong pull towards vernacularisation, that is, an optimisation and accommodation wherein conflicting values and possible courses of action are reconciled such that statements of the 'X is allowed in Y' kind can be made and, moreover, gain currency (Simpson 2013).

However, what we also go on to describe here is the way in which families and individuals, when faced with reproductive crises and dilemmas, also formulate strategies and responses that unsettle presumptions of optimisation. Indeed, some responses do not align with expected audiences and suggest conflict and the possibility that new audiences are featuring in the process of moral reasoning. For example, our interviews revealed instances where consociates in the form of family and community have been actively ignored as individuals choose to work against the grain rather than with it in order to shape their own moral justification and rationale for decision making. These are important dialogical moments in response to ARTs. They are akin to the 'moral pioneering' described by Rayna Rapp in her study of amniocentesis in a US hospital (Rapp 1988,

1998). Her work describes the way in which foetal testing raises novel ethical dilemmas for those presented with the option of testing. She shows how these dilemmas are then worked through by women and men from a variety of class and ethnic backgrounds. The combination of patients' familiar moral beliefs and values brought to bear on wholly novel ethical challenges led Rapp to characterise these women and men as 'pioneers' of a sort, leading the way on behalf of their own communities into unfamiliar and often difficult moral terrain (also cf. Williams et al. 2005).

In the account that follows we present examples of 'addressivity' and 'answerability' evident in the accounts of Pakistani Muslim ART users. We also highlight instances of moral pioneering, triggered, at least in part, by their engagement with IVF. We go on to conclude that moral pioneering may not just be about accommodating new positions in relation to existing values but also aligning with new ones, and particularly the emergence of reproductive privacy as being of primary importance in decision making.

Researching Moral Worlds

The methodological approach we took was in many respects conventional. The fieldwork was carried out mostly among Pakistanis living on Teesside, a heavily industrial conurbation in the north-east of England. The migration of Pakistanis to this region has followed a well-established pattern. Throughout the 1950s and 1960s, single men found their way to the UK ready to fill manpower shortages in manufacturing industries. The remittances sent home did much to alleviate the poverty of the villages they had come from and also enticed others to make the long journey. Many migrants found their way to Teesside, where opportunities in steel, chemical and other heavy industries were widely available and wages were relatively high (Beynon, Sadler and Hudson 1994). Drawn by a nucleus of established male earners, relatives and friends arrived in Teesside, with many coming from the Mirpur region of Pakistan. Throughout the 1960s and 1970s, wives, parents and siblings were brought over and the community consolidated, expanded and 'settled' (Iqbal 2009). It was in this community between 2007 and 2010 that much of our research was carried out.

In the first phase of fieldwork, sixty-five Pakistani women and twenty-three men were recruited from community centres and from 'Sure Start' government centres supporting parents and children with the aim of eliciting views on family formation, infertility and how people deal with it in social and medical terms. In phase two of the study we focused on men and women who had direct experience of infertility treatments (six couples and three individual women). Interviews were informal and wide ranging, and were conducted in English, Punjabi or Urdu, according to respondents' preferences. The snow-balling technique used for this phase of the research took us further afield, with two interviews being conducted by telephone with IVF users resident in London and Bradford. We adopted a life history format, encouraging participants to narrate their marital and reproductive lives in chronological sequence. Participants were reinterviewed after a period of some months, to follow up on new developments in their lives and reproductive careers. In addition, participant observation was carried out in a reproductive health clinic used by the Pakistani community on Teesside, and additional interviews were held with clinicians, embryologists, nurses, social workers and GPs. The materials used in this article are drawn predominantly from phase two of the study, that is, from in-depth accounts of the experience of infertility and the use of ARTs.

Elsewhere we have analysed this dataset in ways that might be thought of as sample-based (Hampshire, Blell and Simpson 2012a, 2012b) – that is, as qualitatively derived data that has the character of separate individuals expressing a view on, or giving an account of, a particular issue. In effect there is a piling up of views to see which vectors are the strongest. This is what Geertz has referred to as 'extensive' data collection and analysis (Geertz 1983). In contrast, the approach we develop in this chapter is ethnographic and 'intensive', and enters into the complex traffic in ideas about culture, identity, continuity, boundaries, remembered pasts and imagined futures that feature in British Pakistani Muslims' accounts of reproductive challenge and its solutions (Hampshire et al. 2014). More specifically we want to understand the ways in which people participate in one another's responses to the predicament of infertility over time, and how their actions and assumptions are shaped with reference to others. Important in this regard was information collected in the four focus groups that we conducted at community centres. On the occasions when contentious topics were raised in these forums it was clear that there was a certain amount of unease about airing discrepant views for an external audience. This public pressure for views to converge around community norms was in contrast to the variability we encountered when discussing issues of infertility and its solutions with individuals and couples on their own. As we demonstrate, the value of an approach that draws on perspectives derived from a variety of settings and circumstances is particularly important where concerns raised fall into the realm of ethics – 'how should I live?' – and, furthermore, in understanding the way that the engagement with ARTs is itself part of a process that enables this question to be posed in the first place.

ARTs and Pakistani Muslims

Amongst Muslims the exhortation to reproduce is well known. In the Hadith, the series of texts that provide commentary and clarification on the Qur'an, it is stated: 'Marry those who can bear children. I will be pleased if you increase the numbers of the *umma* (Muslim community)'. Indeed, the procreative potential of women is seen as integral to their status and the regard with which they are held within Muslim society (Serour 1995). However, as the essential binding agent for a number of ethnic minorities in the UK, Islam is seen as being undermined by a predominantly secular and secularising society. For many, values of familism and procreativity underpinned by religious belief and practice are felt to be under threat and in need of support and preservation (for example, see Bari 2002).

Against this backdrop, the ways in which ARTs are currently being taken up within the Pakistani Muslim community suggest that there is considerable ambiguity: ARTs are welcomed but at the same time they are the object of suspicion and concern. On the one hand, ARTs are embraced because they touch on the powerful and pervasive desire to have children, and offer solutions to a condition that blights public and private lives. In religious terms, the use of ARTs is easily lined up with teachings in the Qur'an that explicitly encourage treatment for infertility (also cf. Inhorn 2003b) and, providing that gametes are taken from a husband and wife, then both Sunni and Shia traditions are broadly permissive when it comes to IVF (Inhorn and Tremayne 2012). This was, broadly speaking, the consensus among our informants, their religious leaders and, importantly, the clinicians they came into contact with who were themselves practising Muslims. ARTs were to be welcomed because, on balance, reproductive imperatives were seen to far outweigh any ethical qualms there might be about helping couples to become parents. As such, ARTs offer a extract, the first woman has raised the issue of IVF in reference to a close relative who is having difficulty becoming pregnant:

> Woman 1: ... because she is not very big, you know, I tell her, ... 'you make a test tube baby' and she says, 'No, my uncle don't like it because in our religion they think it's *haraam*'.
> Woman 2 (interrupting): It's not allowed, yeah, it's not allowed in our religion.
> Woman 1: It's not allowed?
> Woman 2: But some people do, but it's not allowed in our Islam.
>
> [The room gets loud with people's comments]
>
> Woman 2 continues: If we study our Islam, it's not allowed.
> Researcher: Which part is not allowed?
> Woman 1: If they do it with your husband's, you know, his eggs [*sic*], it's all right then God is giving it. But they might make it with some other man's eggs, and give that one, I think.
> Researcher: And that's the problem?
>
> [General agreement]
>
> Woman 1: It's not *halal*.
>
> (Focus group at Women's Centre)

In other words, 'what is most at stake', to use Kleinman's terms (1992: 129) is not so much the practice of IVF per se, but an evident suspicion that 'they' – a predominantly Caucasian and non-Muslim health service – will use other people's gametes to achieve a pregnancy. Notwithstanding such concerns, however, the technologies, if used in accordance with Islam, were accepted by most of our study participants as being a legitimate means to reduce the potential need for adoption, which many felt was a somewhat ambiguous practice within Islam. Most importantly, they were seen to enable couples to avoid the evident catastrophe of childlessness.

Among those interviewed in phase two, however, all had experienced reproductive disruption, and in trying to resolve this problem had engaged more intimately with the moral complexities of IVF in relation to Islam and Pakistani norms regarding families and relationships. For such couples, reflection on these matters revealed tensions and a need to clarify and justify why certain positions were being accepted or rejected. For one man, contemplating ARTs led him to speculate on the relationship between religion and culture and the emergence of a clearly justified position on ARTs. In his view, this position was dependent on education and reference to scripture rather than the vagaries of 'tradition':

> I honestly think it's lack of knowledge really. To be honest with you that's the major thing: my grandparents from my mam's side and my dad's side, they weren't educated ... They were lacking in the knowledge and even with religion, the religion was there but it was more a culture and it was what people said, so that was a major impact as well and with my parents' generation we got more into religion than listening to what our uncle said down the road or what their grandma used to say ... I guess they don't want to make it a public thing; they want to make it a private issue, a private matter because this is where religion and culture and tradition and things get mixed up and some people allow it and some people don't. But religiously that is what we went on and that's what it should be, to be honest with you. It's what people have made up to make religion easy for themselves and really you should be going on religion; it's not hard and everything is written there for you and that's why we got further help from the imams and they actually showed us a couple of verses from the Koran. (H301)

In another instance, the couple had together sought assurances from clerics about their chosen course of action:

> We have read up on the religious side to it and he [husband] has talked to people about it in the mosque and, to be honest, we don't believe it's wrong because as long as it's my eggs and his sperm there is nothing wrong with that. It's only wrong when we start using someone else's sperm or if I use somebody else's eggs – that's when it's wrong; so we are all right with it and hopefully we are doing the right thing. It makes sense as well, and we are both using our own stuff; it's just we are not doing it the normal way how people do it, we are getting help. (W302)

In this case, it is interesting to note that the woman actually raised the question of whether she should pursue IVF treatment at a local community centre and the women there said 'no', it was forbidden (*haraam*); she felt that they were simply not prepared to discuss the matter. The couple reported that they had had more success with their local imam, as well as one consulted back in Pakistan. Both imams reassured them that their actions would not violate Islamic law.

Imams were not the only source of advice when it came to reproductive decision making and Islam. In areas with substantial South

Asian populations, it is likely that some members of the medical profession will also be Muslims and will be known as such by the Muslim community. The couple quoted above readily acknowledged that they used their doctors in this way:

> Not that there is nothing wrong with having doctors from a different religion or a different background, but it just helps when you are the same religion. It helps because if I have a query or there is something I am not sure about, I can go to my doctor as well and I can ask my doctor, 'this is what I am worried about and what is your judgement and your opinion on this', and I've got a choice of that as well, and that helps. (W302)

The doctors we interviewed all shared stories of how they had indeed been called upon to give advice about what steps would be permissible within Islam. Some gave their advice freely and in ways that might be thought of as instituting orthodoxy in the guise of medical practice, while others were more reticent:

> I can't be in both sides: I'm a professional, I just give them a medical opinion. If they need to, they go to their own imam, or whatever … I wouldn't [give an opinion], that is personal. And even if they ask 'are you Muslim?', … I would say 'yes', but 'what is your opinion?' I'd say 'I can't give you, I'm not allowed, it's not my … Even if you ask me in the mosque, if you met me in the mosque and asked me, I wouldn't give you advice because I know you are a patient and I'm a doctor'. I wouldn't. I will pass you to a religious person and then you ask. And I'm sure people appreciate that when you tell them. Because some of them, they come and say, 'We need a donor, we accept a donor'. I say 'That's fine'. 'But is it *haraam* or *halal*?' I say, 'I wouldn't tell you, just go and ask'. (Consultant in reproductive medicine)

At the other end of the spectrum however, some of the more educated and cosmopolitan informants paid little attention to the role of Islam in shaping their decisions. One informant spoke of Islam's 'image problem' and the way in which Islamic conservatives were typically elderly, male and bearded. The idea that they should in any way interfere with private decision making about reproductive matters was thought to be not only inappropriate but reprehensible. She described her relationship with her father, whom she considered 'very Islamic', as a continual source of tension. Her education, independence, choice of a white partner and bearing of children late in life through IVF were all characteristics she felt he considered to be very 'un-Islamic'.

As these examples illustrate, there is often a powerful conjunction of Islamic and family norms that translates into a formidable pressure for Pakistani couples to conceive early in their married life (Hampshire, Blell and Simpson 2012a, 2012b). As the women at the focus group demonstrate, they operate not only with immediate face-to-face relations in mind (consociates) but also, in Schütz's terms, a variety of contemporaries and predecessors. Together these make for influential audiences whose opinions, actual and imagined, play an important role in shaping attitudes and practices where infertility is concerned:

> Woman 1: Our people, they start [gossiping], if you're a little bit late, they start…'
> Woman 2 [interjecting]: It's mainly outside of the family, people are saying 'What's wrong with her, what's wrong with him?'
>
> [The room breaks into loud conversation about this topic.]
>
> Woman 1: The in-laws talk a lot … they say the mother is not healthy. I was very healthy and they were already talking after two months about me not being pregnant. (Focus group at Women's Centre)

The importance of families, and women in particular, in shaping reproductive decision making is further corroborated by a Pakistani GP we interviewed:

> I think you have to convince them sometimes that [folk remedies are] not true and that we should go ahead with the medical treatment. But again, as I said, that influence it comes from the in-laws or their own parents. Mother or mother-in-law has said something … Dad tends to get involved a lot less I think on the fertility side of things I must admit.

And later in the interview:

> Some do [believe in folk remedies], even though they have been born and brought up here. I think it's the parents' influence, the Mum and Dad think that way. What Mum thinks, so that is passed down, but certainly the ones from Pakistan they will have that concept. (General Practitioner)

This familial concern and interest is thus not just confined to relatives in the UK. Reflecting on his visits to Pakistan, one man revealed how questions about offspring tend to be high on people's agenda: 'The first time you go there and you meet the family it will be, "Are you all right? How was your flight out? Do you have any children?" It's the third question' (H301).

Whether for biological reasons or because of conscious decisions to delay parenthood (see also Hampshire, Blell and Simpson 2012a), the evident absence of offspring inevitably becomes the concern of a wider circle of family members, and there is a strong desire to 'please' parents. However, the ways in which these problems might be overcome lead couples into areas of ambiguity and contingency:

> My parents' parents, my grandparents, they were really strict about [marriage] and, to be honest, I don't think they would be happy with us doing the IVF. And my parents, their generation, I think they would think about it, but be two-minded because their parents wouldn't be happy; but obviously with us now it's changing. With each new generation things are changing. (H302)

However, this man's version of gradual but inevitable change across the generations masks some of the tensions that arise on the way. A paradox to which we return later in the chapter is that of a culture of inclusion and intervention among relatives on the one hand and, on the other, technologies that have the potential to redraw the boundaries of public and private life, thereby isolating and separating couples. This issue was again one that exercised the women in the focus group at the Women's Centre, since another option, to avoid drawing in wider family opinions and 'interference', would be to avoid disclosure. As 'Woman 1' said: 'They don't tell anybody; they hide. I tell my auntie, "Do and hide", but she said, "No, your uncle don't like it, he's very strict"'.

But, lest we get carried away with the idea that audiences are always there and have to be taken into consideration, for at least one Pakistani-born couple we interviewed the issue was a *lack* of audience. The burden of the 'pure' relationship – that is, one in which couples make their own decisions on such serious questions – weighed heavily on them: 'Back in Pakistan, there are so many other people like aunties, your dad, your mother; they are caring, but in this country you are a couple [laughs]' (H 204).

Apart from family and community, an important audience for couples is the medical profession itself. As we have already seen, Muslim doctors can play an important role in advising on the morality of certain courses of action. What doctors think is important to couples, even though on occasion the boundaries between technical and moral intervention become blurred. For some patients, this aspect of their intervention was the subject of criticism, particularly where information was concerned. One of our informants (W201) spoke of the 'god complex' in which doctors, typically male, could exercise enormous power over women who were likely to have little understanding of the treatment regimes they were embarking on. This woman described her experiences in a London clinic. The Muslim doctor she was consulting established that she had been sexually active before marriage. In her view, the brusque treatment she received throughout the consultation and the rough handling during a subsequent internal examination was not unconnected to this revelation. In another instance, a woman claimed that, despite her requests for egg donation, she was told that, as she was a Muslim, this was not allowed (W316).

Where language and education were barriers to effective communication between doctors and patients on Teesside, these problems were considerably exacerbated by suspicion about the medical profession. For one couple interviewed, there was an abiding concern about the quality of treatment they had received for the woman's chronic menorrhagia and underlying fertility problems. Failure to address this problem for over a decade gave the man grounds to believe that, as Pakistanis, he and his wife had received inferior medication and treatment from doctors who were corrupt, incompetent and uncaring. His anger and frustration in the interviews was palpable, and brings home the extent to which ARTs require technical and communicational competences as well as moral ones: 'We can't do anything else because we have no money, we have no skills. For these kinds of things you need skills and only me and my wife ... I can't write my name or my address or date of birth ...' (H315).

ARTs and Couples as Moral Pioneers

The emergence of companionate and nucleated family forms among South Asians living in the UK has been documented by a number of researchers (Shaw 2000, 2001; Ahmad, Modood and Lissenburgh 2003; Harriss and Shaw 2009). Education, prosperity and growing acceptance of liberal values has, for many South Asians, led to a growing convergence with wider patterns of domestic organisation and gender equality within the family in the UK. Indeed, normative pressure for what Giddens has referred to as 'affective individualism' is evident in all aspects of contemporary daily life (Giddens

1991; also see Beck and Beck-Gernsheim 1995). In the accounts of reproductive disruption we collected, the engagements with ARTs features as an integral part of this wider trend. Moreover, as we go on to argue, engagement with ARTs is not merely symptomatic of processes of change in this community, it is constitutive of them. It is part of a processual adjustment in which accepted roles and relationships are challenged and changed as couples embark on new possibilities for their domestic and conjugal arrangements. Engagement with ART makes its own contribution to this change as it can bring into question assumptions about patriarchal control and raise questions as to what is choice rather than chance. It also challenges what is thought of as public, private and indeed secret. It is in the context of ARTs that new orientations are set for husbands and wives in relation to what it means to be a couple, and what their mutual expectations might be.

For many of the couples interviewed, their eventual resort to IVF was in some senses prefigured in the choices that had been made earlier in life, and with this came a deviation away from the views of earlier generations (see also Hampshire, Blell and Simpson 2012a). In the following piece of dialogue, it is interesting to note the way that the man interviewed introduces the critical voice of his predecessors.

> Wife: I really didn't want a child at a young age because we know that after two or three years then we would have a baby.
> Interviewer: Did you have that idea?
> Husband: That's pretty much what I wanted as well because I was still at Uni and I didn't have a job. I really couldn't see how we could adjust to a child without having a regular income and I don't want to ask my dad to help out because it's my child; it's not really his responsibility. And that's how I stand as well. ... I think it's more the older people, that generation that are now about sixty or fifty plus, they are the ones bringing from their generations all the ideologies that they have and they are still having, 'You have no children, you have to have children'. But it's like now, when I get to fifty or sixty plus, my outlook on things will be different. I'm different and time changes, doesn't it? Because I see other people who are in their forties and they haven't been saying this and they say, you know, 'You young people take your time, you want to get a bit secure first don't you' and all that, but older people, different age or higher age, they are more, 'No children, you should have had at least four by now' – seriously! [laughing]. (H&W301)

This couple had set themselves against parental expectations of a pregnancy early in marriage but then later found themselves facing unwanted reproductive delay, with resort to IVF the obvious remedy. Similarly, one of the more cosmopolitan IVF users we interviewed put it as follows: 'I think you're kind of conscious of the biological clock ticking, anyway. So for me I'd done my travels, I'd done my career, I'd done my business, you know, sort of aspirations as well. I'd achieved all those things and for me this was my next chapter of my life' (W201).

The respondent was a Pakistani-born woman in her late 30s who had been educated to master's level in the UK and contracted a 'love' marriage. For her, the prospect of 'ostracism' by her family and community held little threat when it came to making decisions about marriage and the timing or methods of family formation. Her use of IVF followed the natural birth of her first child and difficulties conceiving a second at the age of 35. For this couple, using IVF came as part of a wider pattern of options and influences shaping reproductive decision making: the National Childbirth Trust, health and fitness regimes, home-birthing groups, the internet, and consultation with Asian and non-Asian friends and colleagues facing similar challenges of balancing professional and domestic imperatives. Resort to IVF had little to do with any simple fertility drive but was being harnessed with lifestyle and a particular aesthetics of family firmly in mind (see also Hampshire, Blell and Simpson 2012b). It is not surprising to learn that this couple were prepared to countenance the other options that ARTs make possible, such as embryo freezing and egg donation by a sister, in order to have more children at a time of their choosing.

For couples with a more conventional biography, and particularly those who had contracted transnational marriages, IVF was typically used to overcome fertility problems that had delayed early pregnancy. In these cases, the burden of intimacy that ARTs imposed was often greater than for couples who had both grown up in the UK (cf. Charsley 2005). For men in particular, many of the assumptions implicit in the treatment process challenged their ideas of appropriate male roles in relation to women. In a culture that has traditionally attributed reproductive failure to women, a focus on a husband's possible shortcomings was often unwelcome. This response was evident from accounts of some husbands' reluctance to undergo exploratory tests and possibly to receive medication or treatment. A factor here was pressure from in-laws, quick to attribute blame.

> They (in-laws) were putting pressure on me. I thought 'maybe it is something wrong with me' and stuff like that ... so I went to the doctor and I had tests and he goes, 'You're fine', and my doctor, you know, I had him for life and I know him and he said, 'You had tests and everything's fine your bits and bobs are working fine'. They [in-laws] still thought it was me at the time.

Eventually this woman asserted her views about their predicament in no uncertain terms:

> At last I said, 'Right, after this I am not doing crap all'. I put my foot down and told him, I said, 'I don't give a shit what they say'. I said, 'I'm not taking them [the tablets], it's my body'. I said, 'There's nowt wrong with my body – it's you'. And I said, 'I can't even actually tell them – you could'. You know what I mean? You can't really tell them, old people, like that, but I could tell his sister, yeah, but not them. And even then I didn't want to tell her, I never told her ... and I said, 'I'm not taking any more of this crap, I don't care what they say'. Do you know what I mean? ... I'm not, I put my foot down and I said, 'I'm not'. I said, 'Like it or lump it, I'm not, sod off'. I said, 'I know the problem's probably you'.

In this case, the man finally succumbed to pressure from his parents and agreed to have a sperm analysis. She stopped taking the drugs prescribed, and attention turned to the causes of his low sperm count and she later became pregnant naturally.

The reluctance of men to engage with discussions in which they might be identified as the cause of the 'problem' was one that was readily identified by a GP we interviewed who worked on Teesside:

> Usually it's the female who comes in; the males tend not to ... What I have found is that, the male, the kind of ... it's not true that they feel that it's me, you know there is some problem, it takes a long long time for things to ... They find it very difficult, that a man could be deficient of something. They find it very difficult to accept for them that there is something wrong with them, [and] that's why a child can't be born ... Again I think there will be a lot of influence from the in-laws. Mother-in-law, she said to do this and the poor girl will do whatever. Because obviously, one thing is that it's not the male's fault. (General Practitioner)

A desire of some men to opt out of assessment and treatment was often continued into the IVF procedure itself, but here this approach was less of an option, as one of the consultants interviewed opined:

> We do get patients who don't turn up for their appointments but eventually probably their nagging wife will actually tell them to come along, or the consultant ... I mean, we occasionally have a patient who says he's been along to the clinic to produce a sample but when they actually get to the consultation with the gynaecologist, the gynaecologist will find that there isn't any information in the notes ... the patient didn't turn up. (Consultant)

One GP offered his own views on men's poor engagement with the treatment process. Grooms from Pakistan who marry brides from the UK are likely to be at a disadvantage when it comes to knowledge of the processes they undergo, which he put down to basic education in the biology of reproduction. He said: 'Boys who got married to girls from Pakistan who come here, they won't understand; but the girls who were born here certainly understand all right you know, and I think the majority might. Basically they were brought up in this country, the ones I deal with, so they don't have that difficulty I don't think'. This point was echoed by one of our male informants. For him, being educated was key to a complete acceptance of IVF as a solution to their fertility problems: 'Having education it does help and your minds are more broad, and it helps you accept things the way the things work' (H302).

However, acceptance of ARTs and the expectation that couples, not just women, receive treatment unsettles the boundaries between public and private. Amplifying the couple as the locus of primary decision making through joint appointments, information giving, informed consent procedures and an emphasis on confidentiality is likely to set them at odds with a wider audience. As one woman concluded, after reflecting on the likely impacts of family members knowing of her and her husband's predicament:

> Yeah, so he is agreeing that community does have a major impact on a person, on a couple, on whatever decision they do take, and this is why we haven't told many people about it. It's not the fact that we want to keep it private but the fact that it will be harder for us, and people will comment and some people won't accept it, so we have left it between ourselves really. (W302)

By contrast with many other aspects of reproduction within this community, there was reluctance among couples to share the details of IVF procedures, even with close relatives. We might think of this as signifying a change in addressivity; a shift between a situation in which the influence of others is predominant in decision making and the desire to make decisions for and about oneself and each other.

In the South Asian context, Sariola and Simpson refer to this shift as one from heteronomy – rule by others – to a situation of increasing autonomy or self-rule (Sariola and Simpson 2011). This shift also suggests a recasting of secrecy as confidentiality sanctioned by the nature of the biomedical intervention (see Shaw, this volume). Indeed, the expectation that a husband and wife together own their reproductive problems is implicit in the approach of the medical profession when it comes to determining IVF treatment regimes. Both are expected to engage with the treatment and, as we have seen, some couples are entirely at ease with this approach whereas others show great reluctance. What is common to all, however, is a tension between the couple-focused privacy on the one hand and the expectation on the part of kin and community that reproduction is in some sense a public matter. The consequences of making one's reproductive tribulations widely known was brought home by one informant who described how a couple who were known to have finally conceived via IVF after five or six cycles and over two decades of marriage became a running joke amongst their own family members for having had a baby using 'new technology'.

That resort to IVF could result in denigration by those from whom one might otherwise expect support and understanding in part explains the search for new audiences to affirm the validity of actions taken. Couples themselves indicated their solidarity and mutual affection in the face of the pressures that IVF treatment brings. They also indicated the importance of the role of others facing similar difficulties. When asked what might have helped with a difficult and prolonged encounter with IVF treatment, one woman commented: 'I would probably say that maybe there should be some opportunity for parents, prospective parents, to chat to parents who have been through IVF. I am sort of thinking especially [of] those who have twins and thinking about the decision to put two embryos back' (W202). This woman went on to identify the importance of consulting educational materials in books, magazines and on the internet, as well as reference to advocacy and self-help groups such as the La Leche League, a breastfeeding advocacy and support group. Significantly, the emergence of a nascent biosociality (Rabinow 1996) around the experience of IVF and multiple birth was instrumental in her questioning aspects of informed consent in IVF and later refusing the advice of her midwife over supplementary feeding. Moral pioneering, it would seem, not only set her against her own community but also against the medical profession.

Conclusion: Moral Pioneering in Late Modernity

In his classic account of the fate of relationships under the conditions of high modernity, Giddens charted a path along which individuals in contemporary Western societies are drawn (Giddens 1991). Along this route, traditions atrophy and are rejected, and the modern condition becomes increasingly characterised by risk, uncertainty and the illusions of choice and freedom. The thesis is a simple and influential one that has played an important part in charting the transformation of relationships, family and intimacy in late modern societies. However, it has had little to say about ethnic minorities or about the burden that intimacy and reflexivity places on those who find themselves inexorably drawn into it.

In this chapter, we have considered ethnographic and narrative accounts of Pakistanis who, in experiencing disruptions to their desire to become pregnant have resorted to ARTs to resolve these crises. In these accounts are discernible some of the broad outlines of the trajectories that Giddens has written about: the fragility of identities in a pluralistic setting, the move towards de-traditionalisation, the emergence of 'pure' relationships and a growing self-reflexivity focused on the couple as the primary social unit. However, what we have also highlighted are the ways in which ARTs are not merely about individual choices but are rooted in a more complex moral and cultural landscape. This landscape is glimpsed in narrative accounts in which ARTs are the subject of a process of ethical triangulation. Following Schütz, we have identified these points of triangulation in informant accounts of face-to-face relations, as well as beyond these, in an imagined audience of predecessors, contemporaries and successors, all of whom are addressed and occasionally given voice in our conversations. These accounts suggest a delicate navigation between a number of key reference points – imams, the family, the wider community, those 'back home' and the medical profession. The expectations and influences of these people must all be carefully reckoned and, where possible, reconciled with the desire of women and men to become parents on their own terms. In so doing, these couples find themselves acting as moral pioneers in the way that Rapp has described in the case of amniocentesis – that is, persons who, perforce, must fashion new ways of bringing meaning, justification and validation to their use of ARTs to overcome reproductive disruption.

Acknowledgements

This research was funded by the Economic and Social Research Council (RES-000-23-1488). We are also grateful to the couples, doctors and clinicians in Teesside who gave generously of their time to help with the research.

Note

1. The figures in brackets refer to the interview transcripts as they have been deposited in the Economic and Social Data Qualidata archive. The prefix 'W' refers to wives and 'H' to husbands.

Bob Simpson is a professor of anthropology at the University of Durham. His current research interests focus on bioethics, biomedicine and biotechnologies in developing world contexts. An important geographical focus of his work has been South Asia, where he has explored the encounter between challenging technological developments and local systems of values and beliefs. He has also worked on changing forms of kinship and family formation in the UK, and is the author of *Changing Families: An Ethnographic Approach to Divorce and Separation* (1998).

Mwenza Blell is a biosocial anthropologist, and is currently a teaching fellow in the Anthropology Department at Bristol University. Her research concerns biological and biomedical manifestations of social inequality, using innovative methodological approaches to explore biological and social interfaces of bodies in context, and people's own understandings and interpretations of their bodies and experiences. She has carried out anthropological research on a range of topics in the UK, Latin America, South Asia, and East Africa, with a focus on menopause, menarche and IVF. Her current research interests are in gender, intimacy and sexuality, as they relate to embodied experience and biological variation.

Kate Hampshire is a reader in Anthropology at Durham University, UK. Kate is a medical anthropologist and works mostly in sub-Saharan Africa. She is currently working on the use of information and communications technologies (ICTs) and therapeutic technologies (particularly medicines) by children and adolescents in Ghana, Malawi and South Africa. A major methodological focus of her work has been to develop innovative ways of working collaboratively with young people, and to facilitate research partnerships with academics and policymakers in the Global South. She has recently co-edited (with Gina Porter and Janet Townsend) a collection, *Children and Young People as Knowledge Producers* (2014).

ecause not only had he been seen to be fertile, but he had ıcceeded in keeping his lineage intact by using his brother's . Furthermore, this donation had brought him even closer to ɔther.

hsen's case raises several questions ranging from the ethical s of the doctor's action, to the persisting stigma of male infer- ınd the gender dimension of how men and women perceive espond to infertility and its treatment. However, in this er, the focus of the discussion remains on a different aspect of ɔarty gamete donation, namely that of kinship, and the way ıave become instrumental in the hands of infertile individ- vho tend to use them to perpetuate their lineage and forge onds with their kin group, who are the donors or recipients ıete.

ıily and kinship are the foundational sacrosanct institutions ıian culture, acting as guiding principles of social organisa- 'heir significance has not diminished in the face of the major es that have taken place in all aspects of reproductive life in uring the past few decades. Islamic laws and practices, which tensely focused on the protection of family and its perpe- and which define the parameters of relatedness predomi- through biological lineage, further frame and strengthen al values and norms in relation to family kinship. To ensure ntinuity of the family and lineage, pressure on individuals roduce is intense, and infertile individuals are often margin- and have to carry the burden of their barrenness. However, or fertile individuals, reproducing per se is not unconditional ficient to make them welcome, or full members of their kin . The unity of the family being the ultimate priority, those duals who do not have a biological link with the family or n group are rarely welcome members of the kin group.

infertility is such a major stigma, it is understandable that ARTs were first introduced to Iran, a theocratic Islamic they were received with open arms and legitimised in a ely short time, with the full endorsement of leading Shia rs (Tremayne 2009). ARTs' contribution to procreation went urther than just offering a cure for infertility. They became mental in allowing infertile individuals to interpret the rules, gave ARTs legitimacy in the first place, and to use them to heir understanding of what constitutes kinship and to main- ıe integrity of their lineage.

Chapter 3

WHITHER KINSHI

ASSISTED REPRODUCTIVE TECHN
RELATEDNESS IN THE ISLAMIC REI

Soraya Tremayne

I met Mohsen at one of the private IVF clin
me that he had been married for five y
dren, and added, 'My wife is infertile, which
here. With God's will she will conceive'.
positive about his wife's chances of becomi
queried the doctor about Mohsen's optimis
and refrained from commenting, but said 'It
Mohsen yourself'. I returned later to the clin
find that he was leaving without speaking to
expression and a smile on his face. The doct
not wish to talk to you directly, but he kn
rying out research and has agreed that I ca
strict confidence'. The doctor then told me
and not his wife, who was infertile but, o
begged the doctor not to tell his wife the tr
his brother to the clinic to use his sperm to
The doctor had agreed and the fertilisation h
the wife's knowledge or consent. The treatm
and to date she does not even suspect that i
law's sperm that had impregnated her. For

Methodology

The data presented in this chapter are part of a larger study, which started in 2004 and continues to date. The sites of the study are Tehran and Yazd, in Iran, and in the UK, where I worked with Iranian women asylum seekers and refugees. A total of 130 infertile couples were interviewed, one-third of whom remain part of the longitudinal study. The main method used is that of participant observation and in-depth interviews with infertile couples, and the donors and medical personnel, in various public and private clinics. Data in this chapter include the infertile individuals only, and not the donors. In Yazd I worked in the city's oldest maternity hospital, Mojibian, which has a fertility treatment clinic, where I carried out in-depth interviews with infertile couples, through whom I was able to meet a larger number of infertile individuals, and also their wider kin groups. I also had extensive interviews with the leading medical practitioners in the clinic. Thirty-five infertile couples were interviewed, twenty-four of whom were approached in the clinic, and eleven were friends or relatives of those interviewed or were relatives of my host family. In Tehran, between 2004 and 2011, I carried out in-depth interviews with sixty-two infertile couples in three public hospitals, two private clinics and one specialised fertility treatment centre set up to treat infertile war veterans, who had suffered spinal injuries during the Iran–Iraq War. In addition, I interviewed doctors, bioethicists, psychologists and midwives, in and out of the clinics. Through personal contacts, I studied a further ten couples. In the UK, I provided expert reports for courts, for twelve Iranian women asylum seekers who had to flee the country from pending court cases and from extreme violence inflicted on them by their husbands, as a result of fertility treatment through ARTs. The majority of all the cases in the study come from conservative and religious groups in society, with varying levels of education, and a considerable number belong to the middle- or low-income groups.

ARTs, Kinship and Islam

The social and cultural implications of ARTs on family and kinship have been the subject of great interest to anthropologists from the start, and a substantial body of literature exists on them (see, for example, Ginsburg and Rapp 1991, 1995; Strathern 1992a, 1992b; Ragone 1994; Franklin 1997; Edwards et al. 1999; Carsten 2000, 2004; Parkin and Stone 2004). As these studies have shown, the impact of ARTs on family forms and kinship is greater than on any other institution in society. However, views of scholars were initially divided on the impact of ARTs on kinship. For example, Strathern argued that the fact that the users of ARTs have been able to have a choice in the area of human reproduction has 'destabilised' the understanding of kinship, which was perceived as natural rather than socially constructed, in the English worldview. She explained that the availability of these technologies forced the perception of kinship as social construction and as a choice. Susan Kahn's studies of Israel, on the other hand, provided a contrasting example to the argument that ARTs necessarily displace a culture's foundational assumptions about kinship (Kahn 2000: 159). In Parkin and Stone's view, ARTs have resulted in the emergence of 'a tension between kinship as a choice and social construction and the older cultural conception of kinship as rooted in biological reproduction'. Referring to these divergent views, Parkin and Stone (2004: 332) point at a different outcome by stating that although 'new constructions of kinship are occurring in European and American society and in this process choice is playing a larger role, there is at the same time a counter-current drawing Americans back to biogenetic conceptions of kinship'. Inhorn's (2006a, 2006b) and Clarke's (2009) more recent studies of ARTs in the Muslim Middle East throw a different light on what constitutes kinship in Islamic societies. For example, Clarke argues that, '[a]ccording to the vision of the Islamic legal establishments, relations of filiation (*nasab*), are not mutable or fluid, but are given, paradigmatically – but not exclusively – through procreation' (Clarke 2009: 47). Clarke's analysis clearly distinguishes the notions of the Islamic relatedness from the Euro-American ones and its place in relation to the application of ARTs (see also Eich 2012).

Following from the discussions above, the case of Iran provides fertile ground for an examination of whether and to what extent ARTs have dislodged the 'filial' relations by providing a choice for their consumers. In what follows, I argue that the responses of the users of ARTs to third-party gamete donation have evolved from initial resorts to their kin group for gamete donation. Gradually, ART users are moving away from seeking help from relatives and are, wherever possible, secretly resorting to strangers' gametes in order to be able to claim biological parenthood and prove their own reproductive ability.

The history of the legitimisation of ARTs in Iran is well documented (for example, see Akondi 2001, 2006; Inhorn 2003b, 2009, 2012; Tremayne 2006, 2009, 2012; Abbasi-Shavazi et al. 2006, 2008; and Clarke, 2007, 2009). A short overview of this history is that ARTs were introduced to Iran soon after their practice started in the West, and are currently offered in all their forms, from In Vitro Fertilisation (IVF), to third-party donation of sperm, egg and embryo, to surrogacy and sex selection. Stem cell research is carried out too, but is limited in its application. When IVF was first introduced, it went unnoticed by those outside the medical world as it was considered a medical technology and its practice was limited to married couples only. However, with the introduction of third-party donation of sperm and egg, and later embryo and surrogacy, the question of their legitimate practice extended beyond that of the medical sphere and required endorsement from legal and ethical regulatory bodies. In Iran, being a theocracy, the legalisation of ARTs became the responsibility of the leading Muslim scholars, who took a great interest in finding ways of legitimising them, and did so in a relatively short time. As Inhorn and Tremayne (2012), in the context of the role played by religious leaders in the Muslim countries of the Middle East, discuss:

> Initially, these scholars returned to early Islamic texts, in order to examine and better understand the basis upon which kinship and family relations are formed. At first, both Sunni and Shia scholars shared the view that the treatment of infertility and use of ARTs should take place only between a married couple, and that no third party should be involved in this process. The rationale behind this argument was the protection of the purity of lineage (*nasab*), which the intrusion of a third party would destroy and which would lead to biological and social confusion (Inhorn 2003a; Clarke 2009). The effects on kinship and family relations, and the consequent social disorder, were considered profound. (Inhorn and Tremayne 2012: 5)

The Sunni religious leaders therefore banned all forms of third-party donation. Their Shia counterparts, however, subsequently allowed third-party donation, by resorting to independent reasoning (*ijtihad*), which allows senior clerics, faced with new questions, to interpret the Qur'an and come up with new answers. It was the involvement of some of the more liberal religious leaders, who approved of third-party donation, which opened the door for these practices (Inhorn 2006b; Clarke 2007; Tremayne 2009). As Inhorn and Tremayne (2012) explain:

> To understand the process by which ARTs were legitimised with relative speed and ease in Iran, it is necessary to understand two fundamental aspects of Shia Islam: first, the nineteenth-century development of the concept of 'sources of emulation' (*marja'* al-taqlid), or Shia religious scholars who are to be followed for their learnedness; second, the Shia emphasis on independent reasoning (*ijtihad*) to find new answers to arising problems (Clarke 2006). (Inhorn and Tremayne 2012: 8)

Unlike their Sunni counterparts, Shia scholars remain reluctant to engage in formal collective *ijtihad* deliberations on issues of global importance. Instead, they rely on individualistic independent reasoning, which has led to a diversity of opinions among Shia *marajeh*, who, in fact, take opposing views on the interpretation of the Qur'an. Such great scope of opinions has led to considerable 'flexibility' for the Shia *marja* in allowing the introduction of scientific and other innovations. It is the individualistic practice of *ijtihad* that has paved the way for the Shia to engage dynamically with most forms of biotechnology.

Once the use of ARTs was approved by some *marajeh*, the disapproval of other, equally if not more senior *marajeh*, had a minimal impact and remained limited only to the followers of those particular *marajeh*. Besides, many infertile couples, whose *marajeh* did not approve of third-party donation, changed their *marajeh* and joined ones who did endorse it.

In addition to an examination of Islamic texts, the leading Shia scholars also engaged with scholars from other disciplines, such as medical experts, jurists, lawyers, psychologists and bioethicists, to explore the full implications of third-party donation. The history of the engagement of the leading clerics with the specialists is documented elsewhere (for example, see Akondi 2001; Tremayne 2009). The result of these intense debates was that donation of gametes can only take place between a married couple, but a solution was found in the practice of temporary marriage (*sigheh* or *muta* marriage), to legitimise the donation between the donor and recipient of gamete. However, temporary marriage, in this case, did not allow any bodily contact between the donor and the recipient, and the purpose was for the infertile party to legitimately receive the gamete from his/her temporary spouse. The rules also specified that the egg donors should be widows or divorcees, ideally with children of their own, as women could not be married to two men at the same time (Tremayne 2006, 2009). In the late 1990s, Ayatollah Khomeini, the Supreme Religious Leader of Iran, was asked for his opinion on the legitimacy of third-party donation. His approval, which did not refer to temporary marriage, specified that 'donation was allowed as long as no touch or gaze took place'. This endorsement remains open to interpretation to date, but it paved the way for infertile users of gamete to exercise their will in the selection of donors of sperm or egg – a choice that invariably turned out to favour their siblings, or failing this other relatives. While gamete donation by siblings and relatives is practised in many parts of the world (for example, see Roberts 2009), under the Islamic rules this would constitute incest or adultery. Under these rules, men and women are divided into two categories of *mahrams* and *na-mahrams*, which define and determine their social and sexual relationship with each other.[1] The *mahrams* are relatives, who are not potential marriage partners, and any sexual relationship with them constitutes incest. *Na-mahrams*, on the other hand, are potential marriage partners; however, no social or sexual contact or relationship between them is permitted outside marriage. Any transgression from these rules is punishable under the sharia.

The legitimisation of third-party donation, while removing the prohibition of donation between any two parties, raised many questions as far as cultural norms and values and religious and legal practices were concerned. For example, from what precedes, it is clear that when an infertile woman's sister donates her egg and this is fertilised with her brother-in-law's (the infertile woman's husband's) sperm this constitutes adultery, as a man cannot impregnate his wife's sister. The reverse, in the case of an infertile man using his brother's sperm to impregnate his infertile wife, also applies, and both are forbidden (*haram*). However, the infertile parties typically do not see the donation by a close relative in this light. Their understanding of incest and adultery is that of the sexual contact taking place, whereas making an embryo on a petri dish is viewed as a technology, which helps them to conceive[2] (see also Abbasi-Shavazi et al. 2006, 2008). In choosing a close relative as a donor, the ultimate concern is to try and keep the donation 'all in the family', and to avoid mixing one's blood with that of a stranger. In his examination of the significance of 'substance' in Islamic kinship, Clarke argues that, 'for the European or American reader, the substance most naturally associated with the idea of kinship is blood, and Arabic and Islamic concepts are often so translated: *nasab* as 'blood' relationship, for example' (Clarke 2009: 43). Clarke's observations during his fieldwork in Lebanon confirm that blood was commonly used as a symbol of kinship. During my fieldwork, the expression *hamkhouni*,[3] or sharing the same blood, meaning consanguinity, was one that I heard more frequently than any other when donors and recipients used their siblings' gametes and in explaining the reason for their preference for donation from relatives: 'we are from the same blood and flesh and it is obvious that we should help each other maintain our *hamkhouni*'. In their view, the 'best' gamete 'naturally' comes from one of their close relatives. It is clear that 'best' in this case did not mean the healthiest in genetic or medical terms, but implied 'desirable' in that it ensured retaining the continuity of their biological links with their lineage. Interestingly, growing research shows that consanguinity and marriage between cousins or other blood relatives are contributory factors to male infertility, which is transmitted down the male line from fathers to sons. Research also points at the high prevalence of male infertility in the Middle East, where the number of consanguineous marriages is high.[4] Islamic encouragement of marrying one's blood relatives, especially one's first cousins, is a significant contributory factor in perpetuating cousin marriages too. In her seminal book, *The New Arab Man: Emergent Masculinities, Technologies, and Islam in the Middle East*, Inhorn (2012) devotes an entire chapter to what she terms 'consanguineous connectivity' (ibid.: 123–61), in which she explains the prevalence and importance of marrying 'blood' relatives, which is shown to be high ranging between 16 and 78 per cent. Of 220 cases of infertile men, who appear in Inhorn's samples, and who were from various parts of the Middle East, 20 per cent are shown to have married their cousins (ibid.: 137). Cousin marriages are also practised extensively among Iranians, who believe that the Prophet has recommended the marriage between children of two brothers as 'having been arranged in the sky' (meaning in heaven).

To return to third-party gamete donation between close relatives, this form of donation, inevitably, breaks the very rules that allowed it in the first place. For example, on the question of married women not being allowed to donate eggs, most relatives are married and no attention is paid to the rule. Furthermore, if the format of temporary marriage were to be applied in cases of sibling donation, this would be another breach of the *mahram/na-mahram* rules, as a man cannot marry his infertile wife's sister, even temporarily, while he is married to his own wife, to receive the sister-in-law's egg. Nor can a woman receive her infertile husband's brother's sperm. Both cases would constitute adultery.

The degree of closeness is also an important factor in the choice of the donors. Infertile individuals seem to have an order of priority as to who the donor should be. For example, if an egg donor cannot be found among the blood relatives, usually one of the women married to a blood relative is selected. In one clinic, an infertile woman told me 'my husband's brother's wife is going to donate an egg to me. She is married to my brother-in-law and therefore can be considered as a "remote" blood relative'. The terms close (*nazdik*) or remote (*dur*) are often heard in conversation between women in the waiting halls of infertility clinics. The infertile women seem to measure carefully the degree of their affinity with the donor. Some of the women, who had travelled from afar, mentioned that next time they return for the actual treatment they intend to bring their donor who is a *qowm o khish* (*Qowm* denoting the ethnic group, and *khish* the member of the kin group). The implication being that the donor may not be a direct or close relative, but is chosen from among the members of their own kin or ethnic group.

For infertile men too the first choice of donor is their brother. However, one of the interesting aspects of third-party donation is in the way infertile men and women resort to gamete donation. In general, cases of sperm donation do not come to the public attention as much as those of egg donation, as only private clinics practise sperm donation, and in a more discreet way than is the case with egg donation. Similar to the way ARTs have highlighted the persistent kinship preferences among the infertile individuals, they have also made the gender differences, in relation to infertility, strikingly obvious. Male infertility is more stigmatised than female infertility, and men try to hide their infertility whenever possible, as was shown in Mohsen's case. A study by Abbasi-Shavazi et al. (2008) in clinics in Tehran also confirms that infertile men ask their wives to take the blame and claim that they are the infertile party, or face divorce. As I have already discussed elsewhere, even when men resort to sperm donation, especially if the sperm belongs to a stranger, they do their utmost to keep it a secret, so that the child is seen as their biological offspring (Tremayne 2012; also see Abbasi-Shavazi et al. 2006: 383–84 on secrecy). While donations from blood relatives tend to continue, this situation is gradually changing in favour of infertile couples choosing gametes from strangers, as I shall discuss later in the chapter.

Another outcome of legitimising third party donation has been the emergence of donation between siblings of opposite sex, with brothers donating sperm to their sister's infertile husbands (Garmaroudi 2012; also personal communication). This effectively means an embryo formed with a brother and sister's gametes, which, biological and genetic concerns notwithstanding, would be incest from a cultural and religious perspective. The idea of incest, through the practice of ARTs, is not unique to the Islamic world. Edwards' study (2004) of women in the north of England provides an interesting example of the deeply rooted fear of incest. Women interviewed by Edwards were asked whether they would use third-party donation; they replied that they would not because they were not sure whose sperm they would be using. It could be their father's or that of their boyfriend's father or some other relative. As Edwards discusses, what provoked such a reaction by these women was the abhorrence of committing incest by receiving an anonymous donor sperm, which could turn out to be that of a relative. In the case of Iranian recipients of gametes, as mentioned earlier, the two possibilities could not be further apart. Even those infertile couples who were not aware of the religious endorsement did not consider gamete donation an act of incest or adultery, as was also observed by Abbasi-Shavazi et al. (2006). As one woman told me 'this all happens outside my body'.

Finally, in cases of surrogacy, the same pattern of preference for using relatives as surrogates is exercised. In the early days of the introduction of surrogacy, very few women were prepared to act as surrogate mothers, due to cultural constraints, which prevented them from being seen to be carrying another couple's child. At that time, in 2004, only family members were prepared to act as surrogate. Since then, as the practice has become better known, an increasing number of commercial surrogate mothers have come forward, and currently hundreds of women act as surrogate mothers. Once more, it has been the endorsement of religious leaders that has made the practice acceptable in the eyes of their users. However, in her study of surrogacy in Iran, Garmaroudi (2012) shows the strength of the bonds between relatives, who continue to act as surrogate for their kin group, especially the siblings.

The involvement of the infertile couples' kin group does not stop at donation between relatives. Reproduction is still a matter for the entire kin group, especially the husband's side of the family, regardless of whether he is the infertile party or not. The motivation for the man's kin group stems from the fact that he has the ownership of the child, hence his family's greater interest in the matter. In cases of female infertility, often one or more members of her husband's family, the mother-in-law or brother-in-law, accompany her and get involved in discussions with the medical staff. If the husband has an older brother, he lets his older brother take charge of the negotiations with the clinic. I have witnessed scenes in which relatives' tempers rise, rows break out and fists are banged on tables in attempts to make doctors agree to the demands of the family. In one case, reported by Abbasi-Shavazi et al., the infertile woman mentioned that she and her husband were trying to keep the treatment secret from their relatives:

> because every time we go to the clinic, my mother-in-law and sister-in-law telephone me and tell me to be careful that the clinic does not use somebody else's gamete on us. My brother-in-law told us today, that 'you are busy with other matters and are not paying enough attention to what the clinic is doing and they may use another person's gamete for you. Therefore, I am going to accompany you in future, so that you are not cheated'. (Abbasi-Shavazi et al. 2006: 384–85)

Effectively one person's infertility becomes the 'kin group's infertility'.

In addition, the drive for conception is so strong that even those couples who cannot afford the costs of the private treatment try and use the private clinics. This is even more so in the case of sperm donation, a service that the public clinics do not offer. In such cases, relatives may join in to raise the necessary funds, by selling their car or mortgaging their house to pay for the cost of treatment. The financial contribution of the kin group towards the fertility treatment, among other Muslim countries in the Middle East, is also confirmed by Inhorn's study (2012). Through such involvement of the extended families, the clinics, especially the private ones, have encountered regular conflicts arising between relatives, mainly over the ownership of the children born as a result of third-party donation. Some clinics have taken the choice of the donor into their own hands by selecting a suitable donor from their own data bank, and keeping his/her identity confidential from the recipients of gametes. In the process, they inevitably break the very rules upon which the donation has been allowed, namely that the child should inherit from his biological parent. So, as the practice of ARTs continues and new problems arise, the medical practitioners are forced to find new solutions and redefine the boundaries of what is permitted in terms of interaction between the donors and the recipients of gametes. As a result,

ARTs have gradually moved into the realm of medical technologies and are increasingly controlled by the medical practitioners; this means that fewer infertile couples may be able to resort to their relatives for donation in the long run. Interestingly, as ongoing research is beginning to reveal, the unrelenting interference by the kin group at all stages of the treatment is forcing the infertile couples to try and minimise the involvement of their relatives by withholding information from them, and even seeking gametes from strangers to keep the relatives out. But, in doing so, these couples have also realised that once a child is born through third-party donation they can claim to have had their own biological child, and nobody needs to know that they have resorted to using a stranger's gametes. However, this secrecy is not possible for every couple – only those who live in larger cities are able to get away from the daily contact with their close relatives and seek treatment without their knowledge.

The findings of this study have also brought to the fore the gender dimensions of the third-party donation, and the ways men and women relate to a donor child (born from a donor gamete). For women, whether they are the infertile party or not, the process of procreation remains the same. From gestation to breastfeeding, women are able to develop the bonds they need to establish 'real' kinship with the child who is conceived through a donated egg. Breastfeeding itself constitutes the milk kinship, which in Islam is equal to the same rules as the biological kinship. For the infertile men in this study, who had resorted to strangers' sperm, the fact that they played no part in the creation or the gestational phase left them passive and isolated. Their role, as the biological father, had vanished altogether and they considered themselves 'merely' the social fathers. As I have discussed elsewhere (Tremayne 2009, 2012), being merely a social father has provoked a range of reactions among men, from depression to violence. My findings were confirmed through the interviews I carried out with several counsellors and psychologists who had treated these social fathers. However, the real insights into infertile men's behaviour have come from my work with Iranian women asylum seekers in the UK, whose husbands had rejected the donor children and had turned violent towards their wives and children. The data also show that the donor children, who have been conceived through the relatives' gamete donation, had been treated with more warmth and were welcomed as the 'real' members of the family, regardless of the fact that their biological and social parents may have had arguments and disagreements over them. Although information on donor children among the families who have used anonymous and/or strangers' gametes is scant, it is clear that these children, especially if they are the result of sperm donation, had not necessarily brought the anticipated stability to the family (also see Tremayne 2012). However this aspect needs further research.

Conclusion

This chapter started with a case study, that of Mohsen, to illustrate the importance of biological relatedness, and the length that infertile individuals go to ensure the continuity of their lineage. Mohsen's case is not an isolated one, and abundant evidence substantiates the ingrained belief in biological connection, providing the base for family and kinship across the Muslim Middle East (see Inhorn 2006b; Clarke 2009). In this study, the wish of couples to have their own biological child is expressed not only among the infertile cases themselves, but is also confirmed through the examples recounted by doctors and practitioners in the clinics. The introduction of third-party gamete donation in Iran initially provided the perfect solution for infertile individuals. They swiftly realised that not only could these technologies allow them to have children who belonged to their own blood and lineage, but they could also become instrumental in consolidating their bonds with their kin group through the exchange of gametes. In Iran a few years after the introduction of third-party gamete donation, these methods proved the perfect solution to achieving the ideal model of reproduction for the infertile party, in that the secret gamete donation could make them appear as the 'biological' parents of the children conceived through donation. The question arises whether and to what extent, in the long run, the balance of infertile individuals' reliance on their kin group for gamete donation will hold or shift against that of secretly resorting to strangers' gametes. Whatever the choice, the result points to the fact that ARTs 'do not necessarily displace a culture's foundational assumptions about kinship' (Kahn 2004), and indeed they can become the perfect medium in paving the way for infertile individuals to achieve their metaphysical and cosmological ideals of reproduction.

Finally, literature is abundant on the innovative ways that consumers have made use of global technologies to make them fit into local cultural moulds. For example, as Unnithan-Kumar, in her study of female-selected abortion in India observes, 'it is not the technologies that bring about social transformation but it is in how they are made socially meaningful that their power lies' (Unnithan-Kumar 2009: 13). Horst and Miller's (2006) prolific studies of digital technologies in various cultures are further examples, as is the study of the interface between modernity and tradition (Wilkerson and Parkin 2012), which questions 'to what extent traditions themselves are exploiting modernity in creative ways, in the interest of their own further developments'.

Notes

1. Men and women who are related by blood or through fostering, and who are thus not potential marriage partners, are *mahrams*. *Mahram* women to a man include his mother, grandmother, daughter, granddaughter, sister, aunt, grandaunt, niece, grandniece, his father's wife, his wife's daughter (that is, a step-daughter), his mother-in-law, his foster mother, foster sisters, and any foster relatives that are similar to the above-mentioned blood relatives. *Mahram* men to women are her father, grandfather, son, grandfather, brother, uncle, granduncle, nephew, grandnephew, foster brothers, and any other foster relatives (see also Clarke 2009).
2. In the course of discussions I had with various parties at the clinics, there was unanimity that donation of gamete did not hint at any sexual act.
3. On the question of the significance of blood as the substance which constitutes kinship, both Inhorn (2012) and Clarke (2009) have extensively discussed the question of substance in kinship. In this chapter I do not attempt to elaborate on the context of which substance is the basis of relatedness, but refer to the infertile individuals and their perceptions and beliefs of which substance is the basis of relatedness – which in this case is blood.
4. Personal communication from the Head of the Embryology Unit, University of Oxford, UK.

Soraya Tremayne is co-founding director of the Fertility and Reproduction Studies Group (FRSG) and founder of Social Analysis and Anthropology Associates. Her theoretical and research interests include reproduction, kinship, gender, food and ethnicity, and her current research focuses on the politics of reproduction in Iran, with a focus on religion and assisted reproductive technologies. She has carried out research in Iran, Nigeria, Romania, Malaysia and Hong Kong.

Chapter 4

Practitioner Perspective

Practising ARTs in Islamic Contexts

Farouk Mahmoud

As a gynaecologist with a special interest in assisted reproductive technologies (ARTs), a practising Muslim and a scholar who has recently completed a doctoral thesis on Islam and ARTs, the editors of this volume have invited me to provide a brief commentary on the previous three chapters, which have dealt with the way ARTs are being taken up by Muslims in a variety of different settings. Brought together under the heading 'ART Journeys and Moral Pioneers', they provide significant comparative insights into the varying responses of Lebanese, Iranian and UK-based Pakistani Muslims faced with the religious, legal, ethical and cultural implications that an engagement with ARTs inevitably brings. In this commentary, I would like to offer a few brief observations that I hope will provide further illumination of the important issues raised, and that may extend the dialogue yet further.

Clarke's study 'Islamic Bioethics in Transnational Perspective' provides an insightful analysis of Islamic debates on ARTs among the Sunnis and Shia in Lebanon, and how these two communities have responded as the ethics of assisted conception are brought into focus. Although Clarke's chapter is largely restricted to Shia communities, it highlights key controversies surrounding an 'Islamic bioethics', and the way that these are identified and decided upon through *ijtihad*, a process of principled deliberation, as practised by *mujtahids* – that is, Islamic jurists. Clarke illustrates how Islamic scholars, both Sunni and Shia, in accordance with the Islamic policy of eclecticism, enthusiastically embraced medical and scientific innovation. However, as his chapter clearly illustrates, there are significant debates and controversies around how to engage with particular assisted reproductive technologies within the framework and boundaries of sharia, discarding what is inimical to Islam and the Muslim community. In particular, the Shia sanctioning of third-party egg and embryo donation provides a potent example of such contestation, and has been seen by many Muslims (myself included) to be a transgression of this boundary.

From a practitioner perspective, Clarke's observations are illuminating. He draws attention to the tensions that exist between bioethics, as a well-resourced and global academic discipline in its own right, and the place of an 'Islamic bioethics' within this. His comments are timely given the recent writings on the ethical challenges raised by *fatwa*-based evaluation of ARTs. Sachedina has offered fresh insights into this critical but largely ignored dimension of comparative bioethics (Sachedina 2009). While Sachedina considers Islamic jurisprudence or *fiqh* as all important and vital in deliberations concerning ARTs, he draws attention to the extensive conceptual resources to be found in Islamic theological ethics. In effect what Sachedina (ibid.: 25–76) is suggesting is that the literature surrounding *fatwa* needs to be investigated to explore and understand a deeper legal and conceptual reasoning that lies behind the apparent reasons for certain rulings. According to him, the Islamic ethical principles of public interest (*maslaha*), juristic preference of one solution over another (*istihsan*) and what is deemed proper (*istislah*) along with its derivatives – the *qawa'id al-fiqhi* principles of 'no harm is inflicted and neither reciprocated', 'no harm no harassment' and 'necessity overrides prohibition' provide important moral and ethical dimensions of Islamic thought when faced with problems for which there is no clear textual prescription. Drawing on this less visible tradition selectively and appropriately, Sachedina advocates a framework of ART ethics that would facilitate a dialogue between secular and religious perspectives.

A similar view is expressed by Tappan (2012), who points out that clinicians and jurists have been unable to articulate an Islamic bioethics that accounts for the deontological and teleological norms that underpin the status of any particular act. He also quotes Sachedina's critique and analysis of the relationship between juristic rulings and ethics and their respective roles in Islamic bioethics. As he puts it, 'rather than reading ethics as the outcome of legal rulings, ethics grounded in theology should precede (and ideally is reflected in) the *fatwa*' (Tappan 2012).

What Clarke is able to bring out in his comments, and which resonates strongly with the other two essays, is the limits of a purely legalistic attempt at understanding the process whereby workable decisions are arrived at in practice. Tappan concurs with this when he states that despite Islamic law's important, even foundational role, Islamic bioethics cannot be reduced to or equated with the *fatwa*s of jurists. He adds that *fatwa*s alone do not seem to encompass the full scope or range of moral concern in bioethics, or of bioethical reflection on the use of ARTs. Indeed, as a practitioner, it is clear that the term 'Islamic bioethics' has to have a more expansive coverage if it is to operate effectively within governmental and clinical policy.

In raising this issue, Clarke goes to the heart of another concern that runs through the chapters in Part I. Throughout its history, Islam appears to have faced a tension typically cast as one between religion and modernity. As is apparent in many parts of the world today, this tension is absolutely central to the dynamics of the contemporary Islamic tradition. Religious authorities have a relatively high public profile in both perpetuating and dissipating this tension. In their drive to keep up with the times, the long-marginalised and denigrated Shia appear keen to claim greater rationality and flexibility in their brand of Islamic law, a point also well illustrated in Tremayne's contribution.

In this context it is important to understand the more liberal *ijtijad* of the *Mut'azzilite* Sunni and Shia jurists compared to the more orthodox and conservative Sunnis of *Asharite* persuasion. Sachedina comments that, according to the latter, 'Islamic law is a body of practical rules by virtue of the formulations of jurists based on the revealed texts rather than the dictates of their own intuition' (Sachedina 2009: 45). The substantive role of reason propounded by the former hold that, when the solution is not found in the textual sources, man is capable of arriving at a solution by independent reasoning. However, the use of this approach is questionable, even among some Shia scholars. For example, Seyyed Hossein Nasr has argued that:

> Politically, the sharia contains definitive teachings which form the basis of Islamic political theory. In the Islamic view God is the only

> legislator. Man has no power to make laws; he must obey the laws God has sent for him. Therefore any ideal government from the point of the sharia is devoid of legislative power in the Islamic sense. The function of the political ruler is not to legislate laws but to execute them. (Nasr 1994: 1)

The Shia rulings or *fatwa*s may have popular appeal, and be seen as an attempt to combat the perceived 'backwardness' of individual clerics. However, as a practitioner, my concern is that an approach based on the dictates (sometimes indeed conflicting) of individual clerics, however highly esteemed, constitutes an unsatisfactory basis for evaluating ARTs or constructing a sound formula for the practice of a modern Islamic medical ethics. Again Sachedina is instructive:

> All jurist-theologians, whether Sunni or Shia, maintained that without the endorsement of revelation, reason could not become an independent source of moral-legal decisions; and although revealed law can be known through reason ... human intelligence was not capable of discovering the reasons for a particular law. (Sachedina 2009: 32)

He concludes with an important question: 'Can reason discover the divine will in confronting emerging legal-ethical issues without being eclipsed by human self-interest?' (ibid.).

Finally, Clarke highlights the importance of individual reasoning or *ijtihad* in the Lebanese context, in contrast to collective *ijtihad* by assemblies of experts, which conforms to the Sunna recommendation of collective deliberation or consultation (shura), based on Qur'anic passages, including: 'Consult them [community] in their affairs' (Qur'an 3:159) and 'They conduct their affairs by consultation among them' (Qur'an 42:38).

As Clarke demonstrates, the knowledge and competence of Shia *Marjai'a* in analysing contemporary problems through resort to *fiqh* are undeniable. However, Ayatollah Khamene'i and the late Fadlallah's approval of extramarital conception and the former's permissive approach to sperm donation do not, in my view, conform to conventional sharia norms, the principles of Allah's wishes (*maqasid allah*) and sharia as Allah would have wished it (*maqasid-al-Shari'ah*); the same might be said of the late Ayatollah Fadlallah issuing a *fatwa* based on his doctor-friend's views on female masturbation during Ramadan. According to the more conservative Sunni view, these rulings reflect a 'weakness' of individually pronounced *fatwas* that do not explicitly reference the expertise of other religious and secular experts. Recent collective deliberations on ART issues by clinicians with religious scholars, such as the conference organised by Dr Akondi reported by Tremayne (2012), is perhaps a step towards reconciliation, although these still fall short of a more robust *fiqh* academy or assembly of experts from appropriate disciplines.

In a very different approach to the question of how ARTS are taken up in Muslim communities, Simpson, Blell and Hampshire report on the experiences of Sunni Pakistani Muslim couples in the north-east of England who have experienced ARTs. Their accounts provide a vivid picture of the suspicions, frustrations and anxieties of a community who are not only encountering ARTs for the first time but also doing so within the secular and pluralistic frameworks of the British National Health Service.

Essentially there appear to be three broad groups of IVF aspirants in this study, who are likely to be marked by generation and class. The first is the 'conservative', 'traditional' Pakistani woman, probably married to a man from Pakistan, who lacks secular and scriptural knowledge, lacks economic independence and is likely to have picked up a pastiche of ideas from family elders and other sources 'back home' regarding sharia rules. A positive aspect for this group is that they are typically situated in networks that provide encouragement for the couple to seek medical help early and provide continued moral and financial support. So, despite an endorsement of ARTs from local imams, it would still seem that infertile couples in this group were strongly influenced by the older generation, who typically hold more traditional and conservative values. The second group comprises educated couples, well conversant with ARTs and sharia rules via various media including the internet and a variety of scholars. They have the knowledge and money to fend off (at least partially) interference from the older generation and in-laws, and to and organise their family planning to suit their aspirations and ambitions to achieve at least some degree of educational, social and economic independence. Choices about when to have a baby and whether to use ARTs are typically taken by the couple, although still often within the context of wider 'audiences'. The third group, very much in the minority, have no (or very few) qualms about transgressing scriptural proscriptions from the local imam, or, if necessary, obtaining donor sperm, eggs or embryos. Taken as a whole, the study shows a possible shift afoot, in which the generational influence of family elders is on the wane, giving way to the emerging dominance of educated and economically independent couples who make their own choices regarding timing of conception and utilising ARTs.

Despite the stringent monitoring requirements imposed by the Human Fertility and Embryology Authority (HFEA) in the UK, the interviews reveal high levels of suspicion that IVF units may use sperm, eggs or embryos from an outsider to enhance success rates. I wish to emphasise that this is indeed purely suspicion as it is not possible in the UK to procure sperm in this way. Other concerns expressed by Muslims, although significantly not by people who were actual users, included concerns about inadvertent mix-ups of genetic material in the laboratory. There is basis for this concern; this element of human error unfortunately has occurred in the past, though very rarely. The strictness of regulation prevailing in UK hospitals today and the checking and double checking has made this kind of mix-up almost impossible. However, these fears may play a significant role in distorting the work of physicians to deploy ARTs effectively among Muslims.

Among those who had attended the clinics, poor communication and misunderstanding was the basis for one woman claiming not to have grasped the message that overweight women have very poor success rates with IVF. It is indeed true that she would not be eligible for NHS-funded IVF unless she lost weight. Further miscommunication appeared to arise from a lack of basic knowledge of reproductive biology: for example, the male from Pakistan who reportedly showed discomfort when faced with frank and open discussion of intimate and sensitive sexual matters. Such encounters could well be widespread and, as a practitioner, it strikes me that this is an area where careful training is needed in order to help doctors to understand just what the anxieties may be. For example, where there are problems of sperm quality or motility, or even in cases of azoospermia (total absence of sperms in ejaculate), it may be necessary to reassure that this is not a reflection on 'manhood' and the problem could be 'fixed' by intra-cytoplasmic sperm injection (ICSI) following special sperm retrieving techniques. To produce even better results, the ideal 'audience' may well be a forum located in the community, comprising infertile couples (past and present), GPs, Islamic scholars, ART physicians and nurses, and bioethicists, who could provide accurate information and support, and thus put to rest suspicions and fears around deliberate or inadvertent mix-up of gametes.

Finally, it is worth noting an interesting omission from the accounts reported. Despite concern in many Islamic traditions about male doctors seeing and having contact with women's bodies, apparently none of those interviewed had asked for a female doctor. This, in my view, is a step in the right direction; the doctor should be selected for their competence and not their gender, but it remains in practice an area of great sensitivity.

In the third chapter, Tremayne addresses head-on the controversies arising from third-party participation in ARTs in Iran. In particular she discusses how infertile couples are using siblings as donors or recipients of sperm, eggs or embryos. The central concern here is to perpetuate the lineage in order to realise particular kinship aspirations. The backdrop to current problems lies in the fact that, by and large, Iranians welcomed and embraced the liberal interpretation of Islamic scripture and subsequent favourable rulings by some senior Shia scholars. Family and kinship is sacrosanct in Iranian culture, as it is to Muslims more widely. Indeed, protection of family and its perpetuity is one of the foundational principles of *maqasid al-Shari'ah*; however, it is questionable whether obtaining sperm or egg from a sibling or (perhaps even more problematically) from a cousin could be translated as preserving lineage or *nasab*.

In the case of Mohsen, deception certainly 'saved the day' for him, but does his brother's sperm satisfy Islamic criteria for *nasab*, which consists of conception under the umbrella of marriage with the wife's egg, and most importantly the husband's sperm, to preserve patriarchal lineage? In the scholarly view (within all major Islamic traditions), family lineage depends on transmission of genetic material and not on sibling relationships. Islamic attitudes towards adoption exemplify this well: except for identical twins who share 100 per cent of their DNA, other siblings share only 50 per cent. So, in Mohsen's case, quite apart from his deception, particularly to his wife, and the doctor's (in my view) ethical lapse, his child will only have half his genes, and cannot therefore be said to be a proper inheritor of his (supposed) father's lineage. Notwithstanding these arguments against the interpretations being made in the cases described by Tremayne, I find it surprising that sibling donation (as for consanguineous marriages in the Muslim world) is taken with such equanimity. Tremayne quotes that 'marriage between the children of brothers is made in heaven', but there is contrary advice in the Hadith: 'Be choosy for your *nutfa*s (children), whom to marry, for traits do penetrate [along generations]' and here Prophet Muhammad appears to discourage consanguinity (marriage between first cousins). Theocratic Iran, in its endeavour to find ways of legitimising gamete donation, did so by finding 'legal loopholes' (*hiyal* or casuistry). The legitimacy of this strategy remains controversial and is currently the subject of much debate. Shia scholars' engagement with other disciplines resulted in utilising *mut'ah* to validate donation of eggs. As Tremayne points out, this should only be possible if eggs were obtained from widows or divorcees, because a woman cannot be married to two men concurrently. This was overcome by Ayatollah Khamene'i's *fatwa*, which made no mention of marriage, conventional or even *mut'ah*, and opened the doors to sperm, egg or embryo donation even outside the marriage contract; many (including myself) would argue that this is not permitted under Islam (Qur'an 25:54 – 'He has established the relationship of lineage and marriage'). The practice of Iranian couples opting to use siblings or cousins as donors potentially creates a further problem of incest, adultery and breach of *mahram* rules. However, according to the Shia, the first two do not apply because there is no bodily contact or sexual penetration: as one woman remarked to Tremayne: 'It happens outside her body'.

According to Tremayne, clinics in Iran currently use donor gametes from outsiders, particularly sperm, which enables the father to claim parenthood but creates problems of anonymity, family lineage, inheritance issues and lack of medical information of the biological father. The permission for sperm donation is surprising considering that it is proscribed by law in Iran, but resonates with the observation made earlier that the distance between the high-level theological reasoning and the practical ethics of reproduction are often wide. Thus, by acts of omission and commission, I would suggest that Shia scholars have let their rulings slide down a slippery slope by permitting gamete donation under *mut'ah* to operate outside of married couples, and to a wider field of extramarital relations.

The long-term sequel for father, mother and child does not always have a happy ending. As Tremayne points out, for the mother who nurtures the baby in the womb, confinement and breastfeeding are often able to establish a close sense of bonding, which overcomes the need for a genetic connection. However, this is not the case for fathers and, as Tremayne describes, in the worse-case scenario, fathers may reject the child and exert violence towards the rest of the family. The author postulates that the child, when (and if) informed, might also react unfavourably; it would be interesting to acquire data to establish just what does happen in these cases.

Taken together, these chapters reveal some of the complexities faced by infertile women and men, and their families and wider communities, as well as by medical practitioners, Islamic scholars and secular legislators (among others) in negotiating the bioethical challenges that have accompanied the introduction of ARTs into multiple contexts. I have offered some of my own views, not as a definitive 'right answer', but as one particular perspective derived from my long experience of practising medicine in the UK as both a fertility specialist and a practising Muslim. As new technologies continue to throw up new ethical questions, we should not shy away from frank and open debate.

Farouk Mahmoud is a retired gynaecologist and obstetrician who has carried out doctoral research into the ethics of new reproductive technologies in Islamic societies.

PART II

ARTs and the Low-Income Threshold

Part II – Introduction

ARTs in Resource-Poor Areas

Practices, Experiences, Challenges and Theoretical Debates

Trudie Gerrits

The first part of this book was devoted to what might be called the 'intensification' of ART use, and the kinds of 'moral journeys' (of both people and technologies) that are made when ARTs in higher-income settings becomes accessible to wider sectors of – in this case Islamic – populations. This second part focuses on ART 'extensification' – that is, the opening up of new ART centres in countries where previously this was not an option, what Simpson and Hampshire in the Introduction of this book refer to as the 'third' phase in the story of ART provision. Of course, access to these technologies is still very limited in the settings described in the chapters that follow, and assisted reproduction remains – for now – largely the preserve of elites, who formerly had to travel abroad for infertility treatment (Inhorn and Patrizio 2009; Inhorn and Gürtin 2011). As Willem Ombelet argues in the chapter that follows, wider accessibility to ARTs in lower-income countries will almost certainly depend on their greater affordability. Moreover, he argues convincingly that developing ARTs in resource-poor contexts is important from a reproductive rights perspective.

The Sri Lankan case study, reported at the end of this part, gives further insight into the challenges that private practitioners are

Treatment Experiences: Pain, Emotions, Risks, Costs and (Floating) Hope

Using ARTs does not guarantee a successful outcome; on the contrary, an analysis of worldwide data for 2007 showed an average delivery rate from ART treatment of 27 per cent per single started treatment cycle.[1] In addition, the – often prolonged – treatment trajectories generally entail physical pain and emotional disturbances (Greil, Slauson-Blevins and McQuillan 2010; Gerrits 2014). While starting with high hopes, many treatment trajectories end in disillusionment and frustration about all the emotion, money and time invested. This has been reported extensively for people undergoing treatments in the Global North, but applies also – as the case studies in this part show – in lower-income countries.

All three ethnographies in this part report, with different emphases, on women's treatment experiences. The women in Bangladesh, for example, complained about the pain during egg retrieval, their fear of hormonal imbalance resulting from the medication, the uncertainty and psychological distress during the treatment, and the trauma after failed treatment, in a context of low quality of care. In Botswana, women of the 'second generation', with their more bio-centred view were, not surprisingly, more aware and concerned about bodily effects and emotions during and after (failed) treatments compared to the women of the 'first generation'. In Mali, Hörbst observed, initially the women barely spoke about pain or annoyances resulting from treatments, and they did not express any real concerns about treatment procedures or (long-term) bodily risks. At that stage they were mainly focused on achieving a successful pregnancy. After several (failed) treatments, though, her informants too started to talk about their deceptions and depressions; they lost confidence in their doctors and complained about their lack of experience and the low quality of care they were offering (this was also mentioned by Nahar for the Bangladeshi women). In particular, they became frustrated at not having been informed about low success rates and treatment failures. As ART treatments demand a huge financial investment, the distress arising from treatment failure was often aggravated by the failure (as they saw it) of misinvested money.

In this context, it is important to draw attention to the chapter by the Sri Lankan practitioners in which they reflect on the challenges that they – working in the private sector, where 'a competitive atmosphere prevails' – are facing. On the one hand, private practitioners have an obligation to inform the public and their patients realistically about the availability of ART facilities and the range of possible solutions for infertility problems; on the other hand, they have to advertise and promote themselves in the media, as 'any private sector enterprise'. The authors point to the responsibility of practitioners to contribute to the spread of ethically correct information 'in the absence of a regulatory authority with a remit for public understanding of ARTs'. While in Sri Lanka national regulation of ARTs has been put in place, such regulation does not yet exist in most other resource-poor countries, leaving clinic staff the responsibility and power to determine how and to whom ARTs are offered (Hörbst and Gerrits, forthcoming).

The studies in this part provide only a glimpse of users' experiences of ARTs – bodily, emotional, financially – in resource-poor countries. The further expansion of more affordable ARTs in similar contexts needs to be accompanied by studies that trace users' experiences, during and after treatments, successful and failed. These studies should also include assessments of health care practices (such as informed consent procedures and psycho-social support) that aim to make treatment expectations more realistic, and treatments and treatment failures more bearable.

Reproductive Agency versus Social Pressure and Objectification

Worldwide, ARTs have brought a solution for many infertile people and they are seen as a highly desirable, but thus far unachievable, option for many others. While ARTs thus potentially broaden reproductive agency, they have also been heavily critiqued – mainly in the Global North – for the pressure they put on infertile women (and men), who are required to submit their bodies to demanding IVF procedures, in order to 'do everything possible' to get a child (Franklin 1997). The broadening of reproductive agency through these technologies, it was argued, is thus turned into a constraint. Does this argument also hold when ARTs are offered in resource-poor areas in the Global South?

For Bochow, this was the main question she intended to address in her chapter on Botswana's infertile women. In her conclusion though, she remarks that, based on her interview material, it is hard to judge 'where agency turns into constraint'. She found that 'being young, educated and wealthy contributed to people's ability to shape their reproductive lives according to their wishes'. None of her informants expressed that they felt any form of pressure to procure ARTs; rather they saw its use as a good – even the only – option to resolve their problem. Bochow addresses an interesting and important issue. However, it seems to me that the sort of questions that Bochow poses cannot be fully addressed based on interviews and personal accounts alone, for two key reasons. First, such 'social pressures' are not necessarily visible/tangible for the people involved; and second, it may be that the 'second generation' infertile women in Bochow's study may wish to present themselves rather as 'modern' and autonomous decision makers, independent of pressure from others surrounding them.

Hörbst points to a related debate in the social sciences on ARTs, when speaking about 'doing ARTs' (following Cussins 1996). She shows that Malian women are objectified in some ways when undergoing ARTs, while at the same time this objectification is part of their agency in achieving their final aim, namely to have a child. Ortner (2006) referred to this endeavour as the 'agency of projects', that is, the way people attempt to pursue their own culturally constituted projects in a context of (often) vast power differentials. For example, the women in Hörbst's study seem to be prepared to undergo unpleasant treatments and invest considerable money, time and emotions. For them, it is worth the investment, even though for the outsider – as Bochow stated in her conclusion – it may seem to be a very high investment for an only moderate chance of success. The further study of reproductive agency versus social pressure and objectification in context of the expansion of (affordable) ARTs in resource-poor areas is key, as these technologies may have unintended and undesirable effects, such as putting an immense pressure on women to undergo treatments, particularly in environments where high gender inequity prevails.

Transnational Movements and National ART Regulation

Finally, the chapters in this part touch on the complex transnational movements involved in the international ART business. First, the case studies show how, initially, the elite of Botswana, Mali, Bangladesh and Sri Lanka moved to neighbouring countries where ARTs were more developed (like South Africa, India and Singapore) and/or to Europe and the USA to undergo treatments. Secondly, we see the movement of ART experts, travelling *to* African and Asian countries to set up ART clinics (sometimes in the form of satellite clinics) and to train local staff. The mobility of people and techniques goes along with the movement of clinical practices, laboratory skills, ethical notions and so on, which are, to a certain extent, adapted to local situations and conditions (see also Hörbst and Gerrits, forthcoming).

While Palihawadana and Seneviratne correctly observe that ARTs in developing countries are often introduced in the absence of formal regulations, it should not be forgotten that this was also the case when they were first introduced in countries of the Global North. The immense differences in regulations between Western countries – stipulating which treatments can be offered to whom and under what preconditions – show how different societal, cultural, economic, legal, political and religious contexts impact on such regulations. When ARTs travel to contexts that are even more different, it may be expected that regulations become even more diverse. In addition, Palihawadana and Seneviratne raise the question of the extent to which treatments can be regulated in countries where ARTs are mainly offered by private clinics and paid for by the couples themselves, acting as clients purchasing services. These clients may claim levels of reproductive autonomy that only reflect their own acute wish for a child, without necessarily taking into account future implications, in particular for their own offspring.

The regulation of ARTs in most resource-poor countries is still non-existent and constitutes an enormous challenge for the authorities in charge. In particular, this applies to the regulation of the use of third-party material (donor eggs, sperm and embryos) and bodies (surrogates), which is becoming more and more common in such areas (see Hörbst and Gerrits, forthcoming). Who should/will be involved in the elaboration of national regulations and guidelines? Will this be primarily the responsibility of parliamentarians, medical doctors, ethicists and juridical professionals or will the public, patients (or their associations) and other civil society organisations (including religious institutions) have a say as well? And if so, how, through what mechanisms, and to what extent? The global movement of ARTs and their subsequent embedding in national (resource-poor) contexts constitute important and interesting themes of study of ARTs.

Conclusion

Together, the chapters in this section give important insight into clinical practices and users' experiences regarding ARTs in resource-poor countries, and they point to the manifold challenges that clinics and countries are facing in their efforts to extend accessibility to ARTs. Additionally, the studies refer to a number of theoretical notions and debates, which were prominent in the discussion of ARTs when introduced in the Global North – such as stratified reproduction and 'situatedness', reproductive agency versus social pressure and objectification – and which may contribute to the understanding of similar phenomena and processes in the Global South as well.

Finally, these chapters, as indicated throughout this Introduction, suggest many new themes and questions for further investigation, when (more affordable) ARTs become more widely introduced in resource-poor contexts (though these questions do not apply exclusively to such settings). These questions include: What circumstances and factors – other than financial – affect the access to ARTs for women and men? How should informed consent procedures be employed when a couple may not necessarily have a unified reproductive goal? What are the impacts of gamete donation and surrogacy on existing notions of kinship, parenthood and conjugal relations? And the other way round: how do notions of kinship, parenthood and conjugal relationships affect the way ART regulations are shaped? How are ARTs regulations developed and employed? How do people experience ART treatments? How do different packages of quality of care – in terms of provision of realistic information on success rates and treatment risks, and the way psycho-social support is provided – affect people's treatment experiences? What are the short- and long-term implications of failed treatments for the women and men involved? What is the role of the various patient associations and civil bodies in determining the ways that infertility and childlessness is dealt with, at societal level – for example, regarding destigmatisation? What other non-medical initiatives can be developed to support childless people (for example, facilitating adoption), for whom ARTs are not an option (for financial or moral reasons, or because treatments have failed)?

Addressing these and other questions will be crucial for those involved in regulating, providing and improving care and 'cure' for people with fertility problems, such as policy makers, clinic staff and people involved in associations for childless couples. In addition, studies addressing these questions will – by touching on core values and social institutions – give profound insight into what is really 'at stake' for infertile people in these countries, and what is the potential for change at the start of the twenty-first century.

Note

1. ART fact sheet (http://www.eshre.eu, retrieved 28 April 2014).

Trudie Gerrits (MA, PhD) is a medical anthropologist and holds a position as assistant professor in the Department of Sociology and Anthropology at the University of Amsterdam (UvA). Most of her research work and publications are related to infertility and assisted reproductive technologies (ARTs), both in the Netherlands and abroad. Currently she is involved in a comparative study on the appropriation of ARTs in sub-Saharan Africa, for which she did fieldwork in Ghanaian private fertility clinics. Before working at the UvA she worked for five years at the Ministry of Health in Mozambique.

Chapter 5

Global Access to Reproductive Technologies and Infertility Care in Developing Countries

Willem Ombelet

As the power of medical technology advances, more and more difficult questions are raised about what sorts of rights to such technologies people might have, especially in low-income countries. People surely have a right to basic medical care, and, by extension, global access to infertility care should be seen as a fundamental human right, irrespective of socio-cultural, ethical and political differences worldwide (United Nations 2004). Although IVF (in vitro fertilisation) and related procedures have received significant public attention, infertility care cannot be reduced to assisted reproductive techniques alone. Other options are equally important such as a listening ear and psychological support for infertile couples, convincing local health care providers and policy makers to decrease the economic and stigmatising consequences of childlessness, but also the availability of basic diagnostic procedures, easy methods of ovarian stimulation and timed coitus, intrauterine insemination and reproductive surgery.

The level of infertility care differs considerably from country to country. Many variables need to be considered to explain these differences, such as the economic and political situation of the country, the level of education and reproductive health care, state of the facilities delivering medical care including the quality of the hospitals, the available equipment, facilities to perform surgery in case of complications, the level of postnatal care and many others. In this chapter I look at childlessness and infertility in low-income countries, and offer some of my own views and visions for the future.

The Current Situation

The vast majority of childless couples live in developing countries. According to the WHO, there is a silent population of more than 180 million couples worldwide who are facing the consequences of infertility day by day (Rutstein and Iqbal 2004). Infertility care is probably the most neglected and underestimated health care issue in developing countries. Although the negative consequences of childlessness are much more pronounced in developing countries when compared to Western societies, interest of the international community and local health care providers is still lacking (Van Balen and Gerrits 2001; Vayena, Rowe and Peterson 2002; Ombelet et al. 2008a; Van Balen and Bos 2009).

According to Boivin et al. (2007), countries categorised as 'developing' have a twelve-month infertility prevalence rate ranging from 6.9 to 9.3 per cent (ibid.). Substantial geographical differences are noted, and these differences can be explained by different environmental, cultural and socio-economic influences. In sub-Saharan Africa, infection is the cause of infertility in over 85 per cent of cases among women, compared to 33 per cent worldwide (Cates, Farley and Rowe 1985; WHO 1987). Approximately 70 per cent of pelvic infections are sexually transmitted (STIs), while the other 30 per cent are attributable to pregnancy-related sepsis (Ericksen and Brunette 1996). Similarly, many cases of male-factor infertility are caused by previous infections of the male genitourinary tract (Kuku and Osegbe 1989). Both conditions are best treated by assisted reproductive technologies (ARTs), but most infertile couples in developing countries cannot afford ART because the techniques are too expensive and mostly limited to private centres (Nachtigall 2006; Murage, Muteshi and Githae 2011; also see Nahar, Bochow and Hörbst in this volume).

The consequences of involuntary childlessness can be much more severe in developing countries and can create more wide-ranging societal problems than they do Western societies, particularly for women. Negative psycho-social consequences are often intense, and childless women are frequently stigmatised, isolated, ostracised, disinherited and neglected by the entire family and even the local community. This may result in physical and psychological violence and, in some cases, divorce or polygamy (Daar and Merali 2002; Dyer et al. 2004; Dyer, Lombard and van der Spuy 2009; Umezulike and Efetie 2004; Ombelet et al. 2008b). Women tend to be disproportionately blamed for infertility and can be ostracised and assaulted by their families, even driven to suicide or killed. Because many families in developing countries are completely dependent on children for economic survival, childlessness has to be regarded as a major social and public health issue and not just an individual medical problem (Van Balen and Gerrits 2001; Van Balen and Bos 2009; Gerrits and Shaw 2010).

Reduced fecundity in HIV-infected individuals is common (see also Bochow, this volume) and, as a result, marital instability and polygamy may in turn increase the spread of HIV-1 infection (Dhont 2011a). HIV is three times more prevalent in infertile couples when compared to fertile controls in the same population (Nabaitu, Bachengana and Seeley 1994; Dhont 2011a). HIV and infertility share the same determinant of high-risk sexual behaviour. Both conditions are more common in resource-poor countries, may lead to stigmatisation and isolation, and are strongly influenced by socio-cultural and economic conditions. Treatment options are generally expensive, and in both cases the final result is a diminished population. On the other hand, HIV treatment is becoming more effective and available at lower prices, which is not the case for infertility treatment. Awareness, attention, documentation and research of the HIV problem are much more pronounced compared to the infertility problem, which remains mainly hidden. Public solutions are being applied for HIV, while for infertility the solution is mainly found in the private sector. It is striking that budgets for HIV research are huge and the information on HIV is easily available, while the contrary is true for infertility.

Despite well-documented observations of the social and economic consequences of infertility and childlessness in low-income countries, surprisingly little interest is shown in the issue at national and international levels. The two key arguments that are typically put forward to explain this neglect are overpopulation and limited resources.

The overpopulation argument suggests that in countries where overpopulation poses a demographic problem, infertility management should not be supported by the government. It is well known that the world's population is expected to increase from 6.7 billion in 2005 to 9.2 billion in 2050 (United Nations 2007). Between now and 2050, an estimated 35 million people will be added each year to the population of the developing world, and 22 million of them are projected to be in the least developed countries. Therefore, national and international health strategies have tended to focus on reducing total fertility rates (number of children per woman), while infertility care has received little or no attention (Hamberger and Janson 1997).

But even if infertility treatment could be made more accessible in developing countries it would probably account for less than 1 per cent of all deliveries. Increasing efforts aimed at family planning and health education can readily overcome this small contribution to the fertility rate. Denying infertile couples access to infertility care is not a fair population control policy (United Nations 2004). United Nations data not only show that the majority of developing countries have already succeeded in reducing their total fertility rate below 2.5; the data also show that the expected population growth in developing countries is mainly due to an improved life expectancy rather than high fertility rates (United Nations 2007). To illustrate the complexity of the problem further, it is well known that the fertility rate of a specific country is positively related to infant mortality, which is understandable when aged couples are economically dependent on their children in many developing countries (Palloni and Rafalimanana 1997).

According to the 'limited resources' argument, it is hard to justify expensive fertility treatment in settings with few resources and apparently more important health challenges to deal with. Can expensive techniques be justified in countries where poverty is still an important issue and where health care systems still struggle with the huge problem of infectious diseases such as malaria, tuberculosis and HIV? In most developing countries, the reduction in maternal mortality and the promotion of contraception are considered to be the main reproductive health priorities (Aboulghar 2005). Improved 'reproductive health education programmes' have proven to be an excellent preventive tool against overpopulation, sexually transmitted diseases (STDs) and pregnancy-related infections (Okumu, Kamau and Rogo 1990; Lutz and Goujon 2001). But, even with better education and preventative care programmes, involuntary childlessness will remain an important problem for millions of couples.

Reproductive autonomy is the main argument in favour of the provision of infertility treatment in developed countries. The argument goes that people have the right to decide when, how many and how to have children (United Nations 2004). Why should citizens of developing countries not have the right to have at least one child, especially if we succeed in simplifying the methods of infertility care and making these affordable for a much larger part of the population?

To get donor funding for infertility care is nowadays almost impossible. At the Genk Institute for Fertility Technology we recently carried out an internet search for possible donors. A questionnaire dealing with the scope of their actions and the interest in infertility care in developing countries was sent to the most important foundations, NGOs and international societies linked to reproductive health. They all showed interest in the issue of childlessness in developing countries, but in none of these organisations has infertility care been funded before, and no future projects were planned. Considering national governments, it is not only the resource constraint that prevents the provision of infertility services in many developing countries. With the dominant discourse focusing on controlling overpopulation, it is no wonder that infertile women are marginalised and consequently excluded from health sector interventions. Infertile women are victims of the systematic process of 'cultural' exclusion, but in some countries they are also 'institutionally' excluded. Studies show that in a patriarchal society like Bangladesh, where motherhood is synonymous with womanhood, childlessness destroys the identity of womanhood, resulting in marginalisation (Nahar 2012b, see also this volume).

'Men and woman of full age, without any limitation due to race, nationality or religion, have the right to marry and to raise a family'. This statement was adopted sixty years ago at the 1948 UN Universal Declaration of Human Rights and cannot be misunderstood: it implies the right to have access to fertility treatments when couples are unable to have children.[1] At the United Nations International Conference on Population and Development in Cairo in 1994, the following statement was made: 'Reproductive health therefore implies that people have the capability to reproduce and the freedom to decide if, when and how often to do so … and to have the information and the means to do so' (United

Nations 2004). In 2004 the World Health Assembly proposed five core statements, including 'the provision of high-quality services for family planning, including infertility services' (World Health Assembly 2004). The International Federation of Obstetricians and Gynaecologists (FIGO) stated that 'women and men have the right to the highest available standard of health care for all aspects of their sexual and reproductive health' (FIGO 2003).

Political statements and commitments need to result in appropriate actions but progress towards the attainment of these goals on the subject of infertility in developing countries remains slow. The reasons are multiple and include, among others, the problem of 'brain drain', lack of collaboration between politicians and health care providers, budgetary constraints and lack of political commitment (Fathalla et al. 2006). On the other hand, the most important non-profit international organisations, including Family Health International, WHO, International Planned Parenthood Federation (IPPF) and the Population Council, still focus on safe motherhood, the reduction of unsafe abortions, prevention of STDs and HIV/AIDS. The implementation of infertility treatment in developing countries is not a priority for these organisations.

The Future

The level of reproductive health care education is very low in most developing countries despite it being the most cost-effective strategy in the prevention of unwanted pregnancies and sexually transmitted diseases (Lutz and Goujon 2001). A better education is strongly associated with lower fertility rates, and increasing access to education for women is probably the best strategy for an optimal population control (ibid.). Incorporation of reproductive health education into general health education should be a policy supported by governments in developing countries across the world. Data from social science researchers have shown that an important barrier to the use of contraception is the fear of consequent infertility. Family planning and infertility are clearly linked, and should be handled in the same centres. Public education on prevention of infertility includes not only prevention of STDs and pregnancy-related infections, but also lifestyle factors, iatrogenic infertility, environmental pollution and contamination. Education programmes are essential and should be updated.

Prevention of infertility remains the most cost-effective strategy for avoiding involuntary childlessness, particularly in countries with a high prevalence of pregnancy-related infections and STIs (Okumu, Kamau and Rogo 1990; Okonofua 1996). Advantages are numerous: prevention programmes are more cost-effective, they benefit a greater number of people than infertility treatment, and will also improve the health status of women in other ways. Last but not least, prevention programmes can easily be integrated within existing reproductive health and family planning services. On the other hand, when resources are exclusively allocated to prevention programmes, millions of childless couples are ignored because prevention will fail in a substantial number of couples. Whilst I believe that governments should give priority to education and prevention programmes, this should not mean that no money goes to infertility treatment at all, especially if we could make infertility care less expensive and therefore more affordable.

From an ethical and socio-cultural point of view, we have to ask ourselves whether we can justify withholding infertility treatment, including ARTs, in those cases where prevention has failed. The view that overpopulation and limited resources are strong enough arguments for not helping infertile couples in developing countries does not take into account the human rights of infertile couples in general, and their reproductive rights in particular (Vayena, Rowe and Griffin 2002), nor does it take account of the underlying causes of overpopulation. Efforts should be made to reduce the excessive negative social reactions to infertility rooted in pro-natalist policies. Infertility treatment should therefore be part of an integrated reproductive care programme including family planning and contraception, maternal care, and reproductive health. Education, empowerment of women and economic prosperity are the most effective solutions to most problems related to both population growth and infertility. Simultaneously, investments in low-cost interventions are justified (Pennings et al. 2009). Reproductive autonomy, justice and equity underpin our efforts to make ARTs available and accessible worldwide – subject, that is, to political stability and a basic level of medical infrastructure.

Raising awareness is another very important issue and one that should be done with great care. Most important is to focus on changing the existing moral and socio-cultural beliefs such that childless couples are no longer isolated and discriminated against. We will need the media, patient organisations and interested politicians to reach this goal. Obstacles will be numerous and will depend on local socio-cultural, political and religious influences. Providing infertility care in developing countries can only be successful if governments are able to diminish the socio-cultural, psychological and economic consequences of unwanted childlessness. Patient support networks have already claimed the right to equitable access to infertility treatment all over the world (Dill 2007). Patients' voices will be crucial when the issue of infertility has to be discussed with policy makers and health care providers.

In order to implement accessible fertility services in developing countries, the first objective is to simplify the diagnostic procedures (Malpani and Malpani 2002). This can easily be organised in one-day clinics. Exploring a couple's infertility is very simple, reliable and comparatively inexpensive. Moreover, all of these procedures can be performed by a small team of health care providers within a short period of time in an inexpensive setting (Ombelet and Campo 2007).

Implementing low-cost ARTs is only possible if we succeed in simplifying the methods of treatment in such a way that they are still effective and safe, but affordable (Blerkom et al. 2014; Johnson, Cohen and Grudszinskas 2014; Ombelet 2014). The number of scientific papers on simplification of ARTs is growing every year. For the retrieval of oocytes in an IVF programme we should if possible avoid the use of high doses of expensive ovarian stimulation medication such as gonadotrophins, GnRH agonists and GnRH antagonists. The use of clomiphene citrate, a very cheap oral drug, has been proven in many studies to be an optimal alternative, with acceptable results, minimal side effects and a very low complication rate (Ingerslev et al. 2001; Verberg et al. 2009).

Lowering the costs associated with laboratory procedures, namely fertilisation and culture of eggs and embryos, represents another challenge (Pilcher 2006). In 2008, the 'Walking Egg' non-profit organisation was founded. From the beginning, Walking Egg has opted for a multidisciplinary and global approach towards infertility (Dhont 2011b; Ombelet 2013). In the Walking Egg Project we strive to raise awareness surrounding childlessness in resource-poor countries and to make infertility care in all its aspects, including assisted reproductive technologies, available and accessible for a much larger proportion of the world's population (Ombelet 2013). To realise this objective, a number of actions are planned including the following: (1) to raise awareness surrounding the problem of childlessness within (a) the donor community, politicians, funding agencies and research organisations through lobbying and publishing, and (b) the general population through information, education and counselling on infertility and its consequences; (2) to study the ethical, socio-cultural and economic aspects surrounding the issue of childlessness and infertility care in resource-poor countries; (3) to develop new methods of making infertility diagnosis and infertility treatment including ART accessible for a much larger part of the population, by (a) simplifying the diagnostic procedures, (b) simplifying the IVF laboratory procedures, and (c) modifying the ovarian stimulation protocols for IVF; and last but not least (4) to work together with other organisations and societies working in the field of reproductive health to reach the goal of 'universal access to infertility care'.

As part of the Walking Egg Project (Dhont 2011b; Ombelet 2013, 2014), we have developed a new simplified method of IVF culturing, called the 'tWE lab' method. With this new system, specifically designed for low-resource settings, we can avoid the complexity of the use of expensive medical gases, high-tech incubation equipment and infrastructure typical of IVF laboratories in high-resource settings (Van Blerkom et al. 2014). A simple chemical reaction was used to produce CO_2 *de novo*, namely the combination of a weak base (sodium bicarbonate), a weak acid (citric acid) and water. The result is a defined atmosphere that is stable for prolonged periods such that culture medium can be equilibrated in advance of an IVF cycle. Fertilisation and embryo development are observed through the glass vacutainer. Preselection of the embryos to be used for transfer can be done without opening the vacutainers.

The tWE lab system is a closed system intended to enable fertilisation and embryo development to occur undisturbed in the same tube until Day 3, when uterine transfers are done. In this closed system we only used 1,000–5,000 motile washed spermatozoa for insemination of the eggs, with very promising results, which makes this technique usable for a large part of the actual IVF/ICSI population, even if a moderate or severe male factor is involved (Van Blerkom et al. 2014). Up to June 2014 seventeen healthy babies have been born after the use this new simplified IVF method. We calculated that the costs associated of building an IVF laboratory can be decreased by at least 80 per cent by applying the tWE lab system, taking into account that only IVF and not ICSI procedures can be performed.

The ultimate aim of the Walking Egg Project is the implementation of good-quality but low-cost infertility centres in low-income settings, if possible integrated into existing Reproductive Health Care centres. Diagnostic and therapeutic procedures and protocols should be affordable, effective, safe and standardised. Ideally, infertility management should be integrated into sexual and reproductive health care programmes.

It should be noted that effective IVF does not end with embryo implantation, but depends on ongoing care during the pregnancy, delivery and beyond. An important risk of implementing ART in resource-poor countries might be the inability to deal with complications following infertility treatment. Ovarian hyperstimulation syndrome, multiple pregnancies, premature babies and ectopic pregnancies are not uncommon in an ART programme. These complications should of course be avoided if at all possible, but the facilities and knowledge of the staff should be adequate to handle such problems. Reproductive tourism, which sees international clients from Western countries travelling abroad because treatment can be offered at lower prices, has been reported in several countries, including India (Vayena et al. 2009), and may pose a real threat to accessibility and affordability of treatments for local patients.

We also have to realise that, even if universal access to infertility care becomes available, barriers will always remain considerable. In some areas of the world, the use of ART is severely restricted because of religious doctrines (Inhorn 2003b; Serour 2006); in particular, adherents of certain branches of Christianity, Islam and Hinduism (among other religions) have been reported to resist the use of donor gametes (e.g. Bharadwaj 2003; see also Hudson and Culley, Tremayne, Simpson and Hampshire, and Mahmoud, all this volume). However, as several authors in this volume have also noted, the relationships between religious belief and views on ARTs are far from straightforward or homogeneous. Moreover, some patients in non-Western countries may be unfamiliar with the more 'high-tech' forms of biomedicine, which might also raise concerns about using ART (Qiu 2002). Working with and educating traditional healers about the new developments in infertility practice may be an important way forward. Because such healers often speak local languages and operate within locally relevant belief systems, their support and cooperation may be crucial (Bhatti, Fikree and Khan 1999; Stekelenburg et al. 2005; Sami and Ali 2006).

Other Perspectives

Infertility care has to be an essential part of a more comprehensive reproductive health care programme that includes infertility and HIV prevention, family planning and safe motherhood, and a bringing together of prevention and treatment programmes (Sharma, Mittal and Aggarwal 2009). In December 2007, the 'Developing Countries and Infertility' Special Task Force of ESHRE (European Society of Human Reproduction and Embryology) organised an expert meeting in Arusha, Tanzania. Global access to infertility care was the key message (Ombelet et al. 2008b), but this can only be implemented and sustained if supported by local policy makers as well as the international community. Accessible infertility care can only be provided in developing countries if there is political will to support actions for gender equality and women's empowerment through education.

The implementation of new reproductive technologies will require well-organised education and training programmes. Regular audits and systems of accreditation and registration should be implemented in order to maintain appropriate standards of care in all centres involved. The need for funding is crucial and is likely to require input and collaboration from various stakeholders. Funding is needed for the fixed costs of new fertility centres (for example, buildings and equipment), the running services (for example, consumables, medication, medical interventions, and staff salaries), for training the medical, paramedical and administrative staff, and for education of the public, which implies contacts with schools, politicians, traditional healers and the media (Sallam 2008).

I hope that the medical and pharmaceutical industry will also make relevant contributions, such as providing cheap medication and manufacturing basic ultrasound and laboratory equipment at low prices. Socially active philanthropic foundations working in the field of reproductive health have to be convinced about the value of this project, taking into account the growing demand from the developing countries themselves, and the case of equity and social justice. Many international organisations have already expressed their will to participate in this initiative; these include the WHO, ESHRE, IFFS, ICMART (International Society for Monitoring Assisted Reproductive Technology) and ISMAAR (International Society for Mild Approaches to Assisted Reproduction). All these organisations can contribute actively in the realisation of this goal. Table 1 summarises the urgent challenges for the Walking Egg Project.

Table 1: Important challenges for the Walking Egg Project (C. Janisch, 2011, pers. comm.)

A coherent strategy is required
A business plan with clear cost structures must be formulated
Personnel are required for advice, training and implementation
Protocols and management policies must be defined
A 'lead organisation' should be identified to support the planning and design phase
Locations for pilot projects need to be decided
Cooperation between different societies is needed
Organisation of scientific studies in the different pilot countries
Define service packages in order to convince people to donate, knowing exactly what they are paying for
A voucher scheme can be used to improve the quality of services through the development of an accreditation process and enhanced competition among service providers
The integration of family planning, safe motherhood care and infertility services will be crucial
A coherent strategy is required

Conclusion

According to WHO data, more than 180 million couples suffer from primary or secondary infertility. The vast majority of infertile and childless couples are residents of developing countries, where childlessness can lead to isolation and abandonment in many cases. Negative psycho-social consequences are often severe, and childless women are frequently stigmatised, isolated, ostracised, disinherited and neglected by the entire family and even the local community. This may result in physical or psychological violence, or polygamy (Daar and Merali 2002; Dyer et al. 2004; Umezulike and Efetie 2004; Ombelet et al. 2008a). Women are usually blamed for infertility and may be ostracised or assaulted by their families, or even driven to suicide or killed. Differences between the developed and developing world are emerging because of differential availability of infertility care and different socio-cultural values surrounding procreation and childlessness.

Bilateral tubal occlusion due to sexually transmitted infections (STIs) and pregnancy-related infections is the most common cause of infertility in developing countries. Consequently, most cases of infertility are only treatable by using assisted reproductive technologies, which are either unavailable or very costly and only within reach of the happy few who can afford it. Prevention remains the number one priority: not only the prevention of STIs but also the prevention of infertility due to unsafe abortions and deliveries. We urgently need better public education on reproductive health and to raise awareness among health care providers and politicians on the importance of childlessness. Most striking is the almost total lack of interest on behalf of the international community, including socially active public health foundations and non-governmental organisations working in the field of reproductive health.

The time has come to change policies and to realise that access to infertility care is one of the largest emerging fields in global medicine. The immense problem of childlessness in developing countries requires greater attention at national and international levels for reasons of social justice and equity. Keystones in the successful implementation of infertility care in low-resource settings include simplification of ART procedures in order to establish accessible good quality infertility services at low cost. Although reproductive health education and prevention of infertility are number one priorities, the need for accessible diagnostic procedures and new simplified reproductive technologies is very high. The success and sustainability of ART in resource-poor settings will depend to a large extent on our ability to optimise these techniques in terms of availability, affordability and effectiveness.

The Walking Egg Project aims to raise awareness surrounding childlessness in resource-poor countries and to make infertility care in all its aspects, including assisted reproductive technologies, available and accessible for a much larger proportion of the population. By simplifying the diagnostic and IVF laboratory procedures and by modifying the ovarian stimulation protocols for IVF, assisted reproductive techniques can be offered at affordable prices. The implementation of low-cost infertility centres in resource-poor countries, if possible integrated into existing Reproductive Health Care centres, will be a crucial step in reaching the ultimate goal of 'universal access to infertility care'. Infertility is likely to become one of the predominant components of future reproductive health care practice. As evidence-based affordable solutions begin to drive global guidance within both public and private health care system solutions, access to care for the infertile couple will become one of the largest emerging fields in global medicine.

To conclude, I believe that global access to infertility care in developing countries can only be achieved when good quality but affordable infertility care is linked to more effective family planning and safe motherhood programmes. To achieve this goal of universal access to infertility care, only a global project with respect to socio-cultural, ethical, economic and political differences can be successful. After a fascinating period of more than thirty years of IVF, only a small part of the world's population benefits from these new technologies because these techniques are either unavailable or too costly in most developing countries. The time has come to give equitable access to effective and safe infertility care in resource-poor countries as well, and to realise ARTs in their third phase.

Acknowledgements

I gratefully acknowledge Ingrid Jossa for the technical support in preparing this manuscript.

Note

1. For the full text, see: www.un.org/en/documents/udhr/index.shtml

Willem Ombelet qualified in medicine from the University of Leuven, Belgium, in 1979 and completed his training in obstetrics and gynaecology in Bruges and Pretoria, South Africa. He has been the president of the Flemish Society of Obstetrics and Gynaecology (VVOG) (2001–2004) and has, since 2002, been the chairman of the Scientific Committee of that society. He is the coordinator of the Special Task Force on 'Developing Countries and Infertility' of the European Society of Human Reproduction and Embryology (ESHRE).

Chapter 6

Childlessness in Bangladesh

Women's Experiences of Access to Biomedical Infertility Services

Papreen Nahar

It is already well recognised that only the wealthiest residents of developing countries have access to assisted reproductive technologies for infertility treatment (Van Balen and Gerrits 2001; Ombelet et al. 2008a; Van Balen 2008; see also Ombelet, this volume). In response to this inequality, scholars have argued for reducing the cost of infertility treatments, and making available low-tech infertility treatments in developing countries on the grounds of social justice alone (Ombelet, this volume; see also Pennings 2008; Ombelet 2009). Greil, Slauson-Blevins and McQuillan (2010) drew upon work by Kielman (1998) and Okonofua, Harris and Odebiyi (1997), to argue that the basic differences between infertility treatments in developing and developed countries relate to acceptance, utilisation of alternative care systems, and availability. However, the main concern in developing countries is, I argue, probably affordability. For example, in India, treatment cost is identified as a major reason why people do not choose biomedical infertility treatment (Widge 2005; Mehta and Kapadia 2008; Unisa 2010; Madge 2011; see also Palihawadana and Seneviratne, this volume for Sri Lanka). As a result, many infertile people in developing countries still seek the traditional forms of treatment that are available locally (Guntupalli and Chenchelgudem 2004).

Bangladesh is a developing country with a population that is mostly Muslim (89.4 per cent) and mainly lives in rural areas (75 per cent) (BBS 2012). Medical pluralism is a prominent feature of the Bangladeshi health care system, shaping people's chosen treatment for infertility along with other health conditions. Both traditional and biomedical treatments for infertility are available. Traditional treatment is available mainly in the informal private sector, and is popular with poorer people, those in rural areas and in urban slums (Nahar et al. 2000; Nahar 2010). In contrast, biomedical infertility treatment is generally only available in the formal sector, with the main services being provided by biomedical practitioners in the private sector. However, infertility services in the formal public sector are almost non-existent. Only one, the Post Graduate Medical Research Institute, situated in the capital city Dhaka, has opened a separate unit for infertility treatment services, but at the time of the study reported here (2003–2004) it did not yet have sufficient resources to provide appropriate services. As a result, ARTs were only available to a handful of relatively rich individuals and couples through the private sector. At that time, four private clinics in Dhaka were providing ARTs; alongside them, some irregular satellite infertility clinics were being run by Indian practitioners, but the activities of these clinics were mostly kept concealed. As in many other developing countries, the ART industry is a growing phenomenon in Bangladesh. By 2010, just six years after my field research, there were reportedly more than twenty authorised private infertility clinics in Dhaka, where over 20,000 couples had sought treatment and more than 479 babies had been born.

The quality of public hospital services is generally poor in Bangladesh; this was highlighted in Zaman's (2005) ethnographic study in a Bangladeshi hospital, which demonstrated the socio-economic and political reasons underpinning inaccessible, unaffordable and low-quality services in hospital settings. However, apart from the issue of affordability there are also what might be called 'cultural reasons' as to why people avoid biomedical treatment for infertility and resort to traditional treatments and associated beliefs about the causes of infertility. Some prefer the interaction between provider and client that is available through traditional forms of treatment. This may also include a consideration of the gender of treatment providers, a consideration for both urban and rural childless women (Nahar 2010; Nahar et al. 2000). In addition to these factors, current health policy does not recognise infertility as a reproductive health issue, which makes the biomedical option even more inaccessible within the country (Rashid and Dristi 2007; Nahar 2012b).

Elsewhere, I have highlighted the presence of various potential risk factors of infertility in Bangladesh (Nahar 2012b). Despite the presence of these risks, there is hardly any information available on the prevalence or the causal factors of infertility in the country. Unnithan (2010a) has also argued that although the presence of the underlying conditions of infertility is significant, no serious public health attention has been paid to this issue in developing countries. Although, for a number of decades, ART use in developing countries received comparatively little attention from researchers (Berer 1999; Van Balen and Inhorn 2002), recent discussion has focused on how the ART industry is booming in some parts of the developing world, particularly in South Asia and the Middle East (Bharadwaj 2000; Gupta 2005; Inhorn 2005). Additionally, a substantial number of studies have emerged from developing countries themselves in recent years. In the South Asian context the majority of studies on ARTs are conducted in India, nonetheless some research is carried out in Bangladesh and Sri Lanka too. These South Asian studies have focused on policy issues, practitioners' views, quality of care, legislation, cost, ethical issues, and local moral dilemma, as well as involving feminist critics of ARTs (see respectively Chakravarty and Dastidar 1986; Mukherjee and Nadimipally 1996; Bharadwaj 2003; Simpson 2004b, 2005, 2009, 2012; Widge 2005; Mehta and Kapadia 2008; Gupta and Richters 2008; Widge and Cleland 2009a, 2009b; Farouk 2010). In a recent extensive literature review, Greil, Slauson-Blevins and McQuillan (2010) suggest that the infertility studies conducted in developing societies generally represent the experience of infertility from the perspective of community-based studies; studies carried out in clinical settings are confined almost exclusively to the developed world. Gerrits and Shaw (2010), while reviewing social science research on the current practice of biomedical infertility care in sub-Saharan Africa, state that essentially only a handful of studies have addressed the way these treatments are offered, used and experienced.

To date, the way in which women in resource-poor countries experience ARTs has hardly been addressed. This chapter begins to fill this gap by capturing the experience of urban middle-class women in Bangladesh. It focuses attention on childless women who have used ARTs, and contrasts their experience with economically deprived childless women in rural areas who express views about ARTs, despite never having used them. In recounting these experiences and views, the chapter demonstrates how infertility treatment works in the pluralistic medical arena of a resource-poor and predominantly Muslim society like Bangladesh.

Methods

This chapter is based on an ethnographic study that comprises the life histories of eighteen rural poor and eleven urban middle-class childless women aged between 17 and 62. In addition to collecting their life histories, key-informant interviews were conducted with biomedical infertility practitioners (3), and informal providers (6). During the rural part of the study I lived for several months in a village in the central north district of Bangladesh. I developed relationships and networks with people living in ten different villages in the area where I resided. For the urban part of the study, I identified respondents mainly through snowball sampling. Oakley (1981: 58) suggests that a feeling of trust needs to be established between the researcher and those being researched in qualitative research. Being part of the day-to-day life of the rural women, as well as spending several hours with urban women through repeated visits, enabled me to gain their trust. This was vital given that the topic being investigated was of such a 'sensitive' nature. Data collection took place over twelve months during 2003–2004.[1]

Dilemmas in Treatment Seeking

I begin this section by exploring the ways in which ARTs affect the lives of their users, including moral conflicts, the physical and emotional impacts, and the exploitation and economic burdens that they face in using them. Although the urban women I interviewed sometimes moved between the biomedical and traditional sectors whilst seeking treatment for their infertility, they always started with biomedical treatment. Unlike their poor, rural counterparts, the university-educated urban middle-class respondents were more committed to modern treatments than 'traditional' ones. However, a number of urban respondents faced moral dilemmas in using ART, particularly regarding third-party gamete donation, surrogacy and the transfer of embryos in order to have a child. Women basically described two types of dilemma, one originating from Islamic religious belief regarding sexual mores, and the other from the cultural stigma linked with ARTs.[2] For example, Dholeshori, who was aged 33 at the time of interview, had married at the age of 30, and had had one cycle of ART treatment; she subsequently miscarried. In discussion she reported: 'When the sperm is from another man, it seems to me the child will not be ours. I feel uneasy about it'.

Some women chose to undergo treatment abroad, as their perception was that foreign clinics provide better quality treatment than Bangladeshi ones. They may also have travelled for treatment in order to keep the treatment secret from their friends and family. Having treatment abroad can add another level to their concerns because of fears that they may be coerced into accepting a third-party donation from a foreigner. For example, when an American doctor asked Normoda (aged 35, never pregnant, married at the age of 18) about 'hiring a uterus' [surrogacy], she expressed two concerns. First, she considered implanting her husband's sperm into another woman's uterus as almost like her husband having sex with another woman. To her, this already seemed like extramarital sex, which is forbidden in Islam. Second, the fact that the clinic was not in Bangladesh made things more complex still. In her own words,

> What is the meaning of having a baby from another woman's uterus? What kind of mother am I if I don't carry the child in my uterus? Moreover, I was in America. Maybe the child would be from my gene, but at that time I needed to rent a uterus of a foreigner, an American. If I did so, that child would be the child of a foreigner. The most important thing is I was not feeling comfortable to implant my husband's semen in another woman's uterus. It is almost like rape, unethical sex. Maybe this is not a real sexual act, but what is the difference between remarriage of one's husband and having a baby in another woman's uterus?

To her, sexual relations out of marriage and hiring a uterus were all highly immoral. However, although there was some stigma attached to high-tech fertility treatment in Bangladesh, I found that women still opted to pursue this in the hope of conceiving a child. Women often kept their use of ART secret from others for a variety of reasons. First, in a culture where the idea of motherhood is glorified and is closely bound up with ideas of womanhood, having a baby without getting pregnant 'naturally' would impact negatively on the social position of a woman. Even if a woman became a mother following the intervention of ART, she would still be considered 'faulty' and an 'inferior kind of mother', since her motherhood was achieved through 'artificial' means. Social stigma associated with ARTs has been widely reported in South Asian contexts (see, for example, Bharadwaj 2003). Second, in Bangladesh, kinship is highly valued and defined in terms of both a blood bond and a bond through marriage. Any bond that appears to fall outside of these categories does not have a place in local conceptualisations of 'family'. This is particularly vital as caste (for Hindus) and lineage (*bongsho*, for Muslims) play an important role in social life. In such a context, keeping the use of ARTs secret may be the only pragmatic way to fulfil both the desire for parenthood and social expectations. For the same reason, adoption is unpopular in South Asia in general and in Muslim countries in particular. Based on empirical data from Lebanon and Egypt, Inhorn has elaborated on the prohibition of adoption in Sunni Islamic societies, showing that Islam does not countenance the lack of biological connection and inheritance in family life (Inhorn 2006b). She reports that whilst fostering is possible, it is rare in practice. In Bangladesh too, the matter of inheritance of property as per Islamic law influences attitudes towards adoption. There is some fostering taking place in Bangladesh but it is not popular (Nahar and van der Geest 2014). Finally, couples may wish to keep their use of ARTs secret, because of rumours of unethical practices and associated stigma; such practices include the illicit use of third-party gametes. In general it is believed that doctors are in contact with unofficial gamete donors, who are typically poorer people. The doctors are said to collect more than the necessary number of eggs or amount of sperm from one donor for a specific patient, after which they store the surplus for use with others; this is how the doctors save money and time. This practice is possible because no issue of legality exists (at least not in practice) to prevent the sale of these bodily fluids or the purchase of eggs/sperm. This view of body fluids is probably related, particularly among poor people, to the selling of organs and tissues for small and inadequate amounts of money. Blood is commonly donated (in exchange for money). Similarly, ovum/sperm can be transacted with little legal hindrance.

Bodily Harm

The urban women with whom I spoke often complained about the side effects of IVF treatment. Everyone who experienced egg retrieval mentioned the terrible physical pain caused by needles and instruments. They were also subject to painful diagnostic tests and medicines with numerous side effects. To them the 'illness' (infertility/childlessness) itself was not physically painful, but the treatment certainly made it so.

The risk of possible side effects brought on by fertility drugs caused anxiety among the women I interviewed. The side effects mentioned included putting on weight, having irregular menstruation, developing an irritable personality, memory loss and losing concentration. The women were worried about the fact that hormonal treatment might have imbalanced their natural body hormone levels, a concern drawn to their attention by information on the internet. Their major complaint was the physical pain that they had gone through during the treatment, and their repeated visits to the doctor. Shindhu who was aged 40, had never been pregnant, and was married at the age of 26, described the pain as follows: 'I became sick of the long-term treatment. People say that pregnancy is painful, but I am not sure if the pain is more than this treatment. When you have labour pain, people at least see the outcome – you have the baby. But out of this treatment pain you gain nothing, just hope and then loss of hope.' As Shindhu's comments highlight, the outcomes of unsuccessful ART for women are not only physical and moral, but highly emotional too.

Emotional Burdens

The urban women who had used ART expressed the psychological distress they had experienced during the treatment, and the trauma they felt after failure of the treatment. They described their journey as an 'unknown' and 'uncertain' one, where no one knew how long the journey would take or what was waiting for them at the end of this 'road'. Urban childless women described the trauma they felt when a treatment failed after they had spent money, time, physical and psychological energy on it. They felt devastated upon receiving a negative result; consequently they suffered from both 'role failure' and 'body failure', and experienced an acute loss of self-esteem. These women thus felt their bodies were double victims. Normoda (aged 35, never pregnant, married at the age of 18) stated:

> I cried a lot at that time [during the treatment period]. The treatment procedure was physically very painful, I bore all these pains. I went to the best doctors of the USA, which is the most advanced

> country. But then I felt very hopeless. I hardly could sleep at night. There were always streams of various thoughts and memories floating in my mind. ... At one point all our money was exhausted and it was not possible to continue the treatment in the USA. We decided to come back to Bangladesh. After spending seven years of my life just in search of a baby, ruining my husband's business, we returned to Dhaka with empty hands ... we were devastated.

Violation of Privacy

Women's fertility becomes subject to scrutiny by relatives and neighbours after only a few years of marriage in Bangladesh (Nahar and Richters 2011). Rural childless women found it impossible to maintain privacy about their infertility and the treatment procedures they pursued but, as I have documented elsewhere, they were not particularly concerned about this, once the matter of childlessness had been disclosed (Nahar 2010). Conversely, the interviews with urban literate women revealed that they highly valued their personal privacy. However, their use of biomedical infertility treatment interfered with their privacy: it was a challenge for childless women to keep their infertility treatments secret, as an urban respondent explained: 'I used to hide everything from others; I did not want to share the fact that I was incapable of producing a child. I always used to think, "How can I tell people that I do not have children?"' However, women often reported that relatives and neighbours always become suspicious and started making comments: 'Hi, what is going on? Why are you not getting a child?', Podma, a lawyer, aged 40, overheard someone saying. 'The years are passing, so and so's wife is not getting pregnant, she must be suffering from something!' Shindhu, already cited above, stated, 'When you start treatment, it becomes your life, month after month, year after year; you have to go there almost every day. How can you hide it from your extended family, even if they are not living in the same house?'

In general, urban childless women in my study had a greater fear of being exposed as infertile compared with their rural counterparts. For the rural women interviewed, it was virtually impossible to keep any matter secret, given the collective lifestyle they have in the village. For urban women, it was also very difficult to keep their ART treatments private. Their privacy was hampered in three ways throughout the treatment procedure. First, the treatment procedures take a long time, and involve repeated visits to the clinics and diagnostic centres, hospital enrolment and ensuing side effects of the treatment. Second, if the couple need any financial support or loans from their extended family or friends for the expensive biomedical treatment, they need to disclose that they are having the treatment. Lastly, their privacy is violated due to the way that doctors practice, as some doctors attend to more than one patient at a time and, in addition, doctors' waiting rooms are not private. As these women are members of a comparatively small, urban middle-class community, many of them belong to the same social network; concerns about confidentiality were thus heightened.

The Cost of Infertility Treatment

As mentioned earlier, ARTs in Bangladesh are only provided in the private sector and as a result they are very expensive for patients. The life histories collected during this study describe how childless urban women are often prepared to stake the family property in pursuit of their treatment. If in-laws disagree or the husband is incapable of paying for the ART treatment, the woman's parents may help. In many cases they opt for the high-tech infertility treatment instead of buying a property, spending all their savings in the process. Childless women may also sell gold jewellery, received from their parents as a dowry or as a gift from the in-laws on their marriage, in order to fund their treatment. As a last resort, childless couples may take out a personal loan. (For further discussion of treatment costs in the informal sector, see Nahar 2012a.)

Quality of Care Issues

Many urban middle-class women in Dhaka seek treatment for infertility abroad. This occurs mainly for two reasons: one is to avoid what are perceived to be 'low quality' services in Bangladesh; the other is to keep their treatment secret. Five out of the eleven participants in this study had sought treatment abroad, travelling variously to England, India, Singapore, Thailand and the USA. All of them had started their treatment in Bangladesh. Those who could not afford to go abroad to Western countries wanted at least to go to India. The respondents mentioned the following as problems of the treatment process in Bangladesh: non-empathetic treatment, inadequate psychological support, poor counselling, unnecessary repeated investigations/medicine, inadequate management of stress levels, limited information about the process of treatment, risks, poor success rates, unclear cost regimes and poor referral systems (Nahar 2010).

Exploitation in Spiritual Treatment

Although urban women mainly seek biomedical treatment, they also sometimes visit traditional spiritual healers and follow difficult rituals (see also Nahar 2010). The reasons they gave for visiting spiritual healers included the common belief that receiving a child is dependent on 'Allah's will'. Repeated failure of ARTs is also a reason for them to try traditional healing and, unlike biomedical practitioners, traditional healers are said to never give up the hope for pregnancy. As one respondent (aged 35, never pregnant, married at the age of 18) stated,

> After having the unsuccessful [IVF] treatment for a number of years, at one point the doctor had suggested me to remove my uterus for health purposes. ... I thought, maybe if I wait, some medical advancement will take place which will be able to make my uterus active. If I remove my uterus (that is what the doctor had suggested for reasons of my health) now that chance will be totally gone ... also we sometimes see even with a 'faulty' uterus one can go to a spiritual healer [*pir* or *fakir*] and have success, if Allah wishes so.

The above quote highlights the contradictory attitude of the modern urban childless women, and the tendency to view spiritual treatment as a pragmatic choice.

Some spiritual healers arrange special prayers for infertile women. However, these prayer sessions are concealed and shrouded in rumour. Such rumours gained momentum when a popular weekly magazine reported in the mid-1990s on unethical practices of a specific spiritual healer's centre. The rumour was that women were plied with sedative drugs there, and then, once under medication, they were taken to different small rooms in the complex compound, where religious leaders known as *Hujur*[3] oversee healing rites. It was also rumoured that in some instances *Hujur*s hire men to have sex with the clients in order to impregnate them. During my participant observation I visited one of the *Hujur*'s compounds in Dhaka, and I found the process of the treatment to be secretive and quite lengthy, involving a number of what might be seen as suspicious steps. For example, I observed that at one point in the treatment, no friends or family members were allowed to accompany the patient, and the *Hujur* asked the patient to carry out an overnight prayer ritual, inside a labyrinth-like shrine.

Notions Regarding ART amongst Rural Childless Women

Although most rural women are unlikely to ever experience ART, they gather information from various sources about it and hold certain opinions. These opinions come primarily from male family members and local traditional healers, who have more access to the outer world compared with rural women, whose mobility is limited. No IVF treatment is available in villages, small towns, or even tertiary hospitals at a district level. Rural infertile women completely depend on traditional healing in the informal sector. The reasons for choosing the informal sector are pragmatic and not only about resource limitation. Traditional providers and patients share the same cultural beliefs about causal factors, mode of payment, gender of the providers and availability of services (see Nahar 2010). The rural participants of this study had only a very vague idea of the biomedical treatments for infertility that were available in the capital city of Dhaka. Indeed, many rural childless women believed that, in biomedical treatment, women are always injected with other men's sperm (usually that of white males) to produce a baby.

Rural childless women's views of ARTs are influenced by the traditional healers they visit. My interviews with such healers demonstrated that they are extremely sceptical of the effectiveness of biomedical treatments for childlessness. They also believe that ARTs are culturally immoral and religiously incorrect. In a context where rural women's mobility is restricted, it is interesting to note that the denigration of IVF is spread by men within rural communities as well as rural traditional healers, all of whom have access to local towns. By denigrating IVF and referring to it as immoral, religiously incorrect and ineffective, the husbands are able to deflect attention from their inability to afford biomedical treatment on the one hand whilst, on the other, enabling them to propose a remarriage, which is considered to be the ultimate remedy for a woman's childlessness in rural villages. For traditional healers, criticism of biomedical treatment can also be useful, as it allows them to try to restore the popularity of their own treatments, claiming that biomedical treatments for childlessness are anti-Islamic.

Discussion

This study reveals the ways in which Bangladeshi urban middle-class childless women have experienced ARTs, and offers by contrast the views of rural women who have never used such treatments. The experiences reported here are largely negative, and generally have physical, emotional, economic and moral dimensions. A number of authors have already discussed the technological hazards that ARTs bring to women's bodies in Western settings (Renate 1989; Rowland 1992; Thompson 2002). The respondents of the current study also mentioned various physical hazards encountered after going through ART treatment. Inhorn and Van Balen suggest that, 'in Western society, childlessness is often thought of as a medical condition involving defective bodily parts and processes' (2002: 11). Fixing the 'faulty' part of the body is the main focus of ARTs, but this ignores the various side effects of treatment and other aspects of childlessness. Similarly, while discussing ARTs in an Indian context, Gupta (2000) indicated that ARTs may give rise to a series of health complications for the woman and her child, such as hyper-stimulation syndrome, spontaneous abortion or miscarriage, ectopic pregnancy, multiple birth, difficult labour and the need for Caesareans, premature births, low birth weight, perinatal and neonatal mortality, and genetic disorders or defects. Almost two decades ago, Inhorn (1994a) provided an account of the dreadful experiences of Egyptian women of the variety of biomedical treatments for infertility, which were often inefficient and had harmful effects. Later, drawing data from the same Egyptian context, Inhorn (2003c) stated that, because of structural and cultural constraints, infertile people in developing countries rarely receive a positive outcome from IVF treatment. Some authors have analysed infertility and its treatment from a feminist perspective and argued that these technologies pose substantial risks to women's bodies when motherhood is pursued 'at all costs' in order to uphold traditional patriarchal family forms (Rowland 1992; Inhorn 1996; Meyer 1997; Rowe 1999; Rapp 2001; Thompson 2002; Gupta 2006).

A significant body of literature has focused on the psychological impact of biomedical infertility treatment and has identified that many women suffer from emotional problems due to unsuccessful

IVF (Beutel et al. 1998; Holter et al. 2006; Verhaak et al. 2007). Greil, Slauson-Blevins and McQuillan (2010) reported that many studies have indicated that the process of infertility treatment can lead to psychological effects in a high proportion of women, which Boivin and Schmidt (2005) argued could be seen as an 'ongoing emotional process' rather than a series of independent emotional events. The current study also demonstrates the emotional load that ART treatment brings with it.

Several studies have focused on quality issues for IVF treatment in India (Widge 2005; Mehta and Kapadia 2008; Widge and Cleland 2009a, 2009b). The findings of these studies correspond with the experiences of my research participants. For example, infertile women often receive inadequate counselling and a lack of information about the process, risks, side effects, and ultimate cost of the treatment. In similar vein, I have demonstrated elsewhere how, in the experience of urban childless women, biomedical providers of infertility treatment in Bangladesh are 'unsympathetic', and that 'ethical standards' are not well adhered to (see Nahar 2010). Two decades ago, experts argued that high-tech infertility treatments created expectations that were unrealistic, expensive and, in most cases, could not be achieved (Greil 1991; Sandelowski 1991; Forrest and Gilbert 1992). Although, worldwide, ARTs have improved considerably, this account endorses the fact that, in Bangladesh (as in other lower-income countries described in this volume), the situation remains much the same as Forrest and Gilberts' descriptions in the early 1990s. The only available option – private biomedical care – is extremely expensive for clients, who are also faced with a low success rate in return for their unfeasibly large expenditure.

The current study also revealed that the main moral dilemma for those ART users who are religious concerns the un-Islamic nature of third party involvement in ARTs (and particularly gamete donation and surrogacy). However, it is worth noting that expression of this religiosity on ARTs exists in Bangladesh at more of an individual level rather than at state level (Nahar 2010). Although Islam is the dominant religion in Bangladesh, with the majority being Sunni Muslims, the state is not run by Islamic proclamation for various historical, geographic and cultural reasons and, unlike in the Middle East, Islam in Bangladesh is practised in a relatively flexible way (Haq 1976; Amin 1996).[4] There is no official government policy available regarding the use of ARTs. No protests or debates regarding ARTs have been raised by the Islamic leaders in public discourse. In this respect, Bangladesh is rather more like Lebanon, as described by Clarke (this volume). Manuals are occasionally published about Islam and ARTs in Bangladesh. The only written document I discovered during my field research proposed that the biomedical treatment for childlessness was anti-Islamic (Zallum 1997: 26); the argument the Islamic scholar provided was that only God is in the position to create human beings, and so people should not manipulate the process, as it is sinful; however, this is the view of only one particular Islamic scholar, and not a state proclamation. Nevertheless, although Islam does not strictly dictate the type of treatments sought for infertility in Bangladesh, this does not mean that religiosity does not play a significant role in peoples' lives and personal decision making. I argue that the use of ARTs is still subject to moral judgement in a person's social and personal life. However, despite the moral dilemmas raised by ARTs, urban middle-class women (with the economic means to do so) tend to choose ARTs.

Using ART is out of the question for rural poor women, as it is typically way beyond their financial means. However, although they do not or cannot use ART, it was observed that they often have negative opinions regarding its morality. I argue that these notions are typically generated by their kinsmen and by the traditional healers they visit. Rural women depend almost exclusively on the traditional healing system but, in the context of medical plurality, urban middle-class Bangladeshi women also seek traditional solutions at certain points of their treatment pathways as well for various pragmatic and spiritual reasons (see also Nahar 2010). However, it appears they may be vulnerable to various forms of exploitation in this process (see Unnithan 2010b and Inhorn 1994a for discussions of similar forms of pluralistic treatment-seeking for infertility in India and Egypt respectively). Risks of exploitation, moral dilemmas around gamete donation treatment from abroad, and the matter of loss of privacy in biomedical treatment also play into this in the Bangladeshi context.

Conclusion

As argued by several authors (Kahn 2000; Van Zandvoort, de Koning and Gerrits 2001; Simpson 2004a), new technologies introduced in a society always take local meanings and shapes. Inhorn, through her studies in the Middle East, has examined how

ARTs have been received in the Middle Eastern Muslim societies and how they have variously served to influence local social and cultural life. By examining Western reproductive technologies in non-Western societies she has focused on the local–global intersections, and interrogated what was 'local' in an increasingly 'global' world (Inhorn 2003b, 2006b).

Through the ethnographic material presented in this chapter, we can glimpse the ways that urban-based middle-class women in Bangladesh, embarking on an IVF journey, must navigate complex and uncertain moral terrain. This includes accepting low quality and lower efficacy rate treatment or travelling abroad for treatment, innovative ways of arranging money for treatment, fighting with the stigma of treatment, struggling to keep the treatment secret, taking often unknown risks when it comes to some forms of 'spiritual treatment' and, in absence of state-level Islamic proclamation, solving a local moral dilemma of ART in their own way. Despite these difficulties and dilemmas, and the stress encountered in procedures that may be unsuccessful, uncertain and expensive, such women continue to use ART treatment when they can afford to, and many go to considerable lengths to raise the resources required. While some of this is unique to the Bangladeshi context, much resonates with the findings of other studies in resource-poor populations, particularly in the Islamic world (see, for example, Inhorn 2003b on the situation in Egypt). As such, this chapter adds to the global debates and discussions regarding ART in developing-country contexts, and the call for infertility treatment that is of high quality, culturally sensitive and, above all, affordable.

Notes

1. The research gained ethical clearance from Monash University, Melbourne, Australia. The study was funded by International Postgraduate Research Scholarship (IPRS) and Monash Graduate Research School Scholarship (MGRS) of Monash University, and the Amsterdam School for Social Science Research, University of Amsterdam.
2. Sex outside of marriage is strictly prohibited and scrutinised by the community. Breaking this prohibition results in serious social punishment (Rob and Mutahara 2001; Barkat and Majid 2003). This punishment could be overt or covert. Using the same logic, gamete donation and surrogacy are considered tantamount to having sex with someone outside of marriage. This would be the subject of public inquiry and result in punishment and stigma.

3. The literal meaning is 'religious leader', but in this case, one particular religious healer.
4. This is to note that Bangladesh was a province of India until 1947. After the British colonial regime, and due to the rule of division appointed by the British coloniser, a partition took place. Two different countries were established on the basis of religion, namely India and Pakistan. The former Indian province of Bengal was divided into two parts: West Bengal became part of India and East Bengal joined with Pakistan as East Pakistan. The division of Bengal on the basis of religion did not work, because despite their religious similarities, East and West Pakistan were culturally wide apart. East Pakistan was socio-culturally closer to West Bengal. There was also economic inequality between East and West Pakistan, where West Pakistan dominated the economy by exploiting the resources from East Pakistan. Thus in 1971 East Pakistan achieved independence as Bangladesh as a result of the Bengali nationalist movement, through an independence war in which three million Bengali's were killed. Historically, therefore, cultural identity is stronger than religious identity for Bangladeshis. This cultural identity is influenced by the broader Bengali culture, whose centre was West Bengal of India, which is dominated by Hindus.

   Hinduism originated in India. Later, two other religions appeared in the sub-continent, namely Buddhism and Islam. These new religions incorporated many values and practices of the Hindu religion. A vast number of people converted to Islam after its emergence in India during the twelfth century. No wonder, then, that until the eighteenth century most of the literary works of Bengal were based on the Mahabharata and Ramayana, the two ancient Hindu scriptures of the Indian subcontinent (Bhattacharji 1983 [translated]). Therefore the old testimony of India is still relevant for both India and Bangladesh. This also has a great influence on popular culture. The value of motherhood is crucial in South Asia as well as in contemporary India (Gupta 2005). It is also important to mention that aside from cultural or legal aspects, all religions including Hinduism, Islam, Buddhism, Sikhism and Christianity pay high tribute to motherhood (Gupta 2000; Riessman 2000; Bharadwaj 2003). Moreover, during the colonial period, British rulers had influenced the laws and state affairs, which definitely also impacted on everyday culture.

Papreen Nahar is a post-doctoral research associate at the Department of Anthropology, Durham University, and a research associate at the Institute of Health and Society, Faculty of Medical Science, University of Newcastle. Her research interests centre on the socio-cultural, political and gender dimensions of health, particularly in developing countries and diaspora communities.

Chapter 7

Ethics, Identities and Agency

ART, Elites and HIV/AIDS in Botswana

Astrid Bochow

Agency in a Landscape of Stratified Reproduction

In this chapter, I wish to describe the use of reproductive technologies among educated professionals in Botswana, a country in southern Africa. Although there have been significant fertility declines in many countries in sub-Saharan Africa over recent decades, many African countries have been noted for their continuously high fertility rates since the 1960s. Scholars working in societies across the continent have found a pattern in which there is a strong desire for children and a deep anxiety about remaining childless (Hunt 2005). These works emphasise the suffering of women who remain childless as they are highly stigmatised and ostracised by their families and communities (Sundby 1997; Feldman-Savelsberg 1999; Upton 2001). As a consequence, the demand for ARTs has risen significantly in many African countries; however, in 2014 there were only thirty-eight IVF clinics on the whole continent (IVF.net 2014). Moreover, in most lower- to middle-income countries where ARTs are available (like South Africa, Ghana, Nigeria and Kenya) they tend to be concentrated in the private sector and are only affordable to well-off elite or middle class members of society. For the majority of people in resource-poor countries, ARTs are simply unaffordable and therefore out of reach.

Medical researchers have responded to these needs by developing low-cost reproductive technologies and opening fertility centres in countries where demand is high but services are limited and trained staff in short supply. For example, in 2009, the Low-Cost IVF Foundation (LCIF) Switzerland founded three low-cost fertility clinics – one in Sudan, one in Arusha, Tanzania, and one in Cape Town, South Africa. Offering an IVF cycle for about US$300 instead of US$12,000, these clinics make IVF accessible for larger sections of the societies in which they are located (Glausiusz 2009; also see Ombelet in this volume). Studies relating to the social acceptability of ARTs in African societies are still very limited but, by and large, indicate favourable attitudes towards the possibilities that assisted reproduction offers (Hörbst 2006; Ombelet and Van Balen 2010). A study of Sudan's low-cost ARTs in the town of Chatom identified increased risks associated with IVF pregnancies, such as premature and multiple birth (Gaily, Elhussein and Karar 2010: 28). These risks are difficult to handle for parents from resource-poor backgrounds as they involve higher treatment costs. Nevertheless the study by Gaily, Elhussein and Karar noticed positive psychological effects on mothers who conceived through IVF, such as heightened self-esteem.

There is, however, still relatively little anthropological or sociological research on the adoption of ARTs in African societies. Consequently, we know little about the moral or ethical perception of these technologies, people's personal experiences of treatment, how reproductive technologies impact on the quest for fertility, or how ARTs are financed (but see Hörbst 2006, and this volume). The latter question is a particularly important one in low-income countries, where infertility treatments are offered mostly by private clinics that demand high 'out-of-pocket' payment.

The unequal access to treatment using the new technologies invites reflection on Colen's concept of stratified reproduction (Colen 1995: 78). This notion is based on the observation that in stratified societies only some women are able to reproduce or fulfil their reproductive desires, while others are bound to take care of the children of others. In some societies, for instance, older women may take care of the mother and the newborn infant (Harcourt 1997). In societies that are highly stratified economically, these carers are typically maids on low income who raise the children of those with higher income (Colen 1995). ARTs intensify these differences and, when viewed from a global perspective, produce a form of stratification whereby people in wealthier regions in the Global North have more and better access to reproductive services than those in poorer countries (Inhorn 2002, 2007b). Transnational connections are an expression of global inequalities. An extreme example of such inequalities is to be found in women offering surrogacy services in India who carry to term the babies of wealthy but infertile couples from the Global North (Kroløkke 2012). 'Reproductive travel' therefore cements the inequality between Global North and South, but may also create a new axis of dependencies between developing countries with a market for ARTs, such as India, and countries in the North where access to reproductive services might be limited due to cost or to laws and regulatory systems that restrict the use of reproductive technologies (Whittaker 2009; Inhorn 2011).

Projecting the anthropological critique of how ARTs reflect global inequalities onto the local situation in Botswana reveals how some women and men are more able to fulfil their reproductive wishes, while many others have little capacity to do so. Yet, as biomedical technologies become available more widely, what does this mean for Botswanan women's (and men's) ideas about fertility and infertility? We know that efforts to limit or induce fertility were widespread in Africa long before the arrival of biomedicine (Bledsoe 2002; Johnson-Hanks 2002). Biomedicine treats infertility as a physical rather than a socially or spiritually induced phenomenon. It sidelines explanations of infertility as being caused by spiritual and cosmological imbalances (Jacobson-Widding and Van Beek 1990; Muller 1999) or as resulting out of social friction and envy, for instance between in-laws and young wives (Feldman-Savelsberg 1999). Instead, biomedical treatments diagnose physical causes for infertility (for example, poor ovulation or ovarian malfunction) and offer a variety of ways to overcome these (for example, gamete donation). In short, the body is seen as being composed of a set of parts and processes that can be artificially acted upon if they 'fail' to perform correctly (Woliver 2002: 39). Franklin has referred to this conception of fertility as the 'make-ability of life' (Franklin 1995). As biotechnologies heighten the potential to manipulate the body and form it according to individuals' needs and wishes, they also require individuals to play a more active role in determining the future of their health. As such technologies begin to appear in places like Botswana, we may see significant changes in the degree of agency and control that people feel over reproductive processes, and their ability to remedy infertility and plan their futures.

The availability of these technologies may also introduce new constraints and pressures, especially for those who enjoy middle-class status but are not particularly rich. In an article on women who go through IVF treatment in the UK, Sarah Franklin (1997) discussed the concept of choice in relation to their striving for fertility. Franklin argued that what appeared at first glance to be a woman's 'choice' to pursue IVF treatment could become effectively a necessity. Childless women who desired children felt compelled to try, and keep trying, reproductive technologies, even though the 'take home' success rate was only between 15 and 20 per cent. If they succeeded, so the argument goes, they would have reached their goal of parenthood and family life. If not, they could at least be satisfied that they had done everything possible to pursue their goal. Franklin's article points out that broadening reproductive agency through reproductive technologies can in fact turn into a new kind of oppression, namely the submitting of one's body to the difficult procedures of IVF in order to 'do everything possible' to fulfil one's reproductive role. The question is what does it take people to fulfil their reproductive desires – financially, socially and physically – and how far do people go to meet these? In what follows I describe and discuss how the availability of ARTs have changed reproductive agency in contemporary Botswana, in particular among the professional classes.

Fertility and Fertility Care in Botswana

The take-up of ARTs by educated professionals in Botswana arises out of the country's increased wealth following the large-scale extraction of diamonds in 1975. This rapid increase in prosperity has brought about tremendous social change, not least in relation to family planning practices and the use of biomedical services. Botswana has become one of the few middle-income countries in Africa, and the lifestyles of its growing number of educated professionals are often cited as an example of the continent's newly emerging elites (Werbner 2004). The country, with its two million inhabitants, hosts a cosmopolitan and educated elite, which is in itself quite diverse and stratified in terms of ethnicity and social background. While, at the beginning of the twentieth century, cattle were the major source of income and wealth, in present-day Botswana these are more likely to come through education. Old political elites made up of chiefs have been replaced by those working in the governmental administration and as civil servants.

Infertility appears to be a pressing problem among educated professionals in Botswana that has some historical depth in a society that places a high value on fertility. Anxieties about infertility were recorded much earlier by the anthropologist Schapera ([1940] 1971) who conducted research among the Tswana-speaking groups in south-eastern Botswana. Schapera described how, in a society where men often had to spend long periods in the mines in South Africa away from their wives and children, children born out of wedlock did not evoke serious moral concern as women were expected to 'make best use of their fertility' (Schapera 1971: 127). Delius and Glaser (2005) offer a similar perspective; where fertility is of high importance in relational ethics, 'sexuality' received comparatively little moral attention. In contrast, educated professionals have been having smaller numbers of children since the 1930s. Instead of large families of up to ten children, they were inspired to have two to four children, depending on their financial capacities.[1] However, despite reductions in family size among elites, having children continues to be of great importance. As I go on to show, childless women in the elites often experienced stigma and social exclusion.

The desire for children gains further urgency in view of the fact that fertility rates are affected by the high prevalence of HIV/AIDS in the country. Botswana has one of the highest HIV/AIDS infection rates in the world. The HIV/AIDS impact surveys released in 2001, 2004 and 2009 estimated the prevalence rate to be 30 per cent in the adult population (Ministry of Health 2001, 2004, 2009). In these surveys, the prevalence rate of women in the age group of 30 to 34 is estimated to be about 50 per cent. Epidemiologically speaking, HIV/AIDS impacts a person's biological capacities to conceive and give birth to children in various ways. For example, weakening the immune system makes the body more vulnerable to other sexually transmitted infections which are known to cause infertility. In addition, women with an unfulfilled desire for children may engage in unprotected sexual intercourse and therefore are exposed to a higher risk of contracting venereal infections, as well as HIV (Dhont 2011a). The result is that populations with high HIV/AIDS infection rates are exposed to a higher risk of infertility. Infertility, just like HIV/AIDS, is a highly stigmatised condition in Botswana. The silence that exists around infertility is quite similar to that surrounding HIV/AIDS. It is also accompanied by shame and humiliation for those affected. Asking somebody about her or his condition is likely to be taken as shaming. In addition, both infertility and HIV/AIDS are related to issues of sexuality and relationships, and are also accompanied by very particular rules about how to talk and not talk about them (Lambert 2001; Arnfred 2004; Geissler and Prince 2007).

Botswana's public health system offers very little assistance for men and women who are infertile. Family planning services do not offer counselling and, despite Botswana's otherwise comparatively well-functioning public health service, it offers only very basic infertility treatment and diagnostics tools such as ultrasound and a hysterosalpingogram (HSG).[2] Although some public hospitals cooperate with private health services, for instance in the use of laboratories, patients often go through a time-consuming system of referrals. Private clinics offer more services, but these are also limited. In 2010 there were fourteen private gynaecological clinics in Botswana's capital, Gaborone. Two gynaecologists, Dr Music and Dr Eaton, practised at the Gaborone Private Hospital and the Bokamoso Private Hospital. The latter opened in 2010 on the outskirts of Gaborone and offers various diagnostic facilities. However, only hormonal treatments and artificial insemination are available for patients in Gaborone; patients who wish to conceive through IVF or ICSI need to go to specialised clinics in South Africa. In Gaborone only one gynaecological clinic, the Gynae and Care Clinic, is specialised in the diagnosis and treatment of infertility. The two gynaecologists working there have been trained in Leipzig, Germany. They offer artificial insemination and will arrange treatment in a fertility clinic in South Africa for their IVF patients, and supervise them before, during and after the treatment. Interviews conducted in 2009 and 2010 indicated that one IVF cycle costs between 40,000 and 65,000 (Botswanan) Pula (3,100 to 5,000 GBP). In summary, fertility care is more available to those who can afford to pay the bills of private gynaecologists; even then, the use of ART is restricted to those who can afford the expensive treatment as well as the additional costs of travels to South Africa and accommodation there.

Sample and Methods

I recruited respondents in Gaborone's private fertility clinics, especially in the Gaborone Private Hospital and Bokamoso Private

Hospital. I also recruited with the help of a pastor of a Pentecostal church as well as counsellors and psychologists. Altogether I collected the reproductive histories of seventy women and fifteen men during three visits to the field in the years 2009, 2010 and 2011. Interviews were conducted mostly in public spaces, cafes and restaurants, and lasted between forty-five minutes and two hours. During the conversations, I took notes, as most respondents did not feel comfortable with recording, and later I produced transcripts based on these notes and my memory. Twenty-five of the women and three of the men I interviewed had sought medical assistance in order to conceive. Their ages (and therefore also their chances of conceiving) ranged from 28 to 55.

The women and men were of different socio-economic status within the group of educated professionals. Their life stories reflected not only the diverse pathways into educated middle class and elite groups in the second half of the twentieth century but also quite different attitudes and experiences towards medical interventions where infertility was evident. Their different experiences and attitudes were not only influenced by differing ethical approaches towards sexuality, relationships and having babies but also by the development of fertility medicine itself and the growth of the medical sector in Botswana. The diversification of the medical sector took place partly under the pressure of the HIV pandemic, which made increasingly sophisticated health care necessary. On the basis of this historical background, I identify two different generations in my sample: the 'first generation' were in their prime fertile years in the 1990s, when fertility medicine was almost non-existent in Botswana; this group also witnessed the arrival of the HIV pandemic. These were women who are today in their late forties to mid-fifties; most are approaching, in, or have passed menopause. What I refer to as the 'second generation' are women who are today in their prime fertile years; their ages vary from late twenties to late thirties.

The interviews I conducted resembled the intimate chats that urban women are used to. They reveal how women express themselves about topics such as biomedicine, health, relationality, professionalism and kinship, depending on which aspect of their history they wish to emphasise. However, this is but one layer of interpretation. When women and men talked about their reproductive lives, neither I nor they had their medical records to hand. For my part, access to medical records was not granted by the research permit I obtained from the Ministry of Health or from the hospitals approached. This resulted in limited knowledge of the biomedical causes of infertility among the women with whom I spoke, and especially where their infertility was as a result of an HIV infection. Some women, particularly of the older generation, remained vague on the causes of their infertility. A very good example is Sophia (see below), who gave a somewhat confusing account of medical treatment and diagnoses.[3] Non-healing infections, however, were recurrent in the medical history she narrated. She also reported that her ex-husband had been HIV positive, as did another informant called Nikki (see below). Taking these two indicators together, it was likely that both Sophia and Nikki were not only infertile but also HIV positive. Throughout the interviews, women of this generation referenced HIV/AIDS, albeit tacitly. The younger generation on the other hand did not reference HIV/AIDS at all. Considering the high prevalence rate, which is close to 50 per cent in their age group, they might well have also been HIV positive.

Pioneers of Fertility Care: Transnational Travel and Fertility

The first generation of women I interviewed about their medical journey had little option to seek treatment for their infertility. By the beginning of the 1980s, Botswana's health system was in a period of diversification. During that time there was only one gynaecologist in the country, working in the Lutheran Hospital in Ramotswa. The National Hospital in Gaborone hired a gynaecologist in the mid-1980s. Gynaecology focused on meeting the demands of childbirth, and there was simply no extra capacity to meet the needs of those who remained childless.

The biographies of those I interviewed from this generation underline the lack of medical expertise for infertility during this period. The first woman I wish to introduce here is Gorata, aged 48, who comes from a family that was already well established in the 1990s. Being part of an early wave of elites, she did not receive her university training abroad and stayed in Botswana for most of her life. Throughout her reproductive life, she suffered from menstrual pain and heavy bleeding. She consulted a general practitioner at a clinic in the mines where her husband worked, who transferred her to a specialist in South Africa. When she consulted him, she was examined but did not receive any diagnosis. The clinic in the mines hired expatriates on good salaries and she trusted that the specialist in South Africa was counted among the best in his profession. Knowing that she had seen the best specialists she did not seek further medical advice. At the age of 40, she was still childless and decided to have her uterus removed in order to avoid further menstrual pain (interview in Gaborone, 12 March 2010).

Some women of this generation had travelled abroad for their education. Nikki, who was aged 52 at the time of the interview, and Sophia, aged 47, illustrate this point. I never met Nikki in person but had a long telephone conversation with her during my time in Botswana. She was first confronted with her fertility problem in Botswana, where she suffered a miscarriage. She started bleeding and lost the baby. She sought treatment at Princess Marina, the National Hospital in Gaborone, where a cyst was found on her fallopian tube. Whilst living in the United States, she visited a gynaecologist specialised in fertility medicine for the first time. Throughout the years, she visited gynaecologists every now and then and tried IVF twice, although without any success. She did not conceive during the time of her marriage, nor after. During her marriage she suffered from violent outbursts from her husband, and ultimately her marriage failed because of her infertility. She later began a relationship with an American who was determined to make her pregnant but eventually she stopped seeing fertility specialists. Nikki received most of her fertility treatment in the United States, where she spent fifteen years (phone interview, 21 November 2010).

The second interviewee, Sophia, described how she travelled to the UK for educational reasons. As she recounted her history, it became clear that her times in the UK were not only times of studying but also times during which she learned more about her own fertility. Now 47, and thus a few years younger than Nikki, Sophia started to narrate her history of infertility by telling me about a miscarriage at the age of 29. By that time she had been receiving Clomid treatment.[4] During her miscarriage she, like Nikki, went to Princess Marina where she received care. However, in the twelve months after treatment she became ill and frail. After this year of illness, she went to a private gynaecologist for the first time. He conducted tests but did not find any problems, and gave her painkillers. By the end of that year she was selected for a training programme as a laboratory assistant in the UK, and left the country. She was happy to leave her life in Botswana behind as she was having marital difficulties at the time. During her one-year training programme she went to a gynaecologist who diagnosed an unhealed infection as the cause of her condition. She was given antibiotics, and the infection healed. Her narrative was marked by long passages in which she talked about her cheating husband and their painful quarrels, and family pressures concerning their relationship as well as their childlessness. She continued fertility treatments in Botswana, where it was discovered that her fallopian tubes were blocked. Soon after that she again left for the UK, this time to enrol in a degree programme. It was in the UK that she sought treatment from a specialist who offered her IVF treatment. However, she did not undergo treatment. Back in Botswana and equipped with a new knowledge, she became a patient of the Gynae and Care Clinic. In view of her age, however, she was advised not to undergo further IVF. Nevertheless, at the time of the interview she was saving for the costs of an IVF cycle in South Africa while at the same time being treated for a new infection in her fallopian tubes (interview, Gaborone, 21 November 2010).

Each of the three biographies represents different ways of climbing up the social ladder. For Nikki and Sophia, travel abroad opened up new options for diagnosis and treatment (although in both cases their reproductive problems remained unsolved), while Gorata, who was from an influential family, stayed in Botswana and had not been exposed to more advanced forms of fertility treatment. In contrast to Gorata, Nikki and Sophia's social mobility was achieved through emigration. Nikki belonged to a group of educated professionals even before her travel to the United States. Her time there gave her access to a diaspora community of artists and intellectuals, who formed the backbone of the political-intellectual elite in Botswana and South Africa. Sophia, by contrast, was of modest rural background, had received state-sponsored education and was never part of elite political circles. At the time of interview, her position had enabled her to obtain a loan to buy a car. The loan was a benefit of working in the public sector and allowed her to enjoy certain middle-class privileges, although the car itself was comparatively modest in contrast to those of other women interviewed. Most importantly, she could not pay for her IVF treatment out of her pocket and needed another loan. Nevertheless, Sophia represents a pioneer who not only used her travels to enhance her social position through education but also used the medical knowledge abroad to seek a solution for her fertility problem at home. Taken together, their travels abroad enabled women of this first generation not only to advance socially but also to use advanced reproductive technologies. In contrast, elite women in that generation who did not travel, like Gorata, had no access to advanced infertility care.

Even though their childlessness was a factor that shaped their biographies, all three women were vague concerning the diagnoses, the courses of treatment and the different specialists they visited. Even when prompted, Nikki and Sophia did not reflect much on how they could have used different therapies to achieve their reproductive goals. And, although they sought biomedical treatment, they devoted little thought to their physical condition. When I went through the notes of my more-than-two-hour talk with Nikki, I was surprised how little information I found on the actual cause of her infertility in contrast to the very detailed information about her education, jobs and relationships, despite my continuous questions on the medical history. It was as if the physical aspect of infertility escaped from her narrative, including the IVF treatment she had received. The same was true of Sophia's biography. At a certain point the emphasis of her narrative shifted away from 'infertility' to her disastrous marriage. These contrasting ethnographic accounts each point to infertility as a cause of marital conflicts and even violence (cf. Feldman-Savelsberg 1999). Indeed, it was not infertility that troubled her during her marriage but rather her husband's extramarital affair. Herein, her story resembled that of many other Botswanan women of her age. In her biographical accounts she emphasised social aspects of suffering, namely the relationships to her (by the time of the interview) HIV-positive husband, a theme that other women with HIV-positive husbands repeated.[5]

It is likely, then, that the women interviewed suffered from both infertility and an HIV infection. Their accounts suggest that these women's travels enabled them to seek medical care for infertility as well as HIV/AIDS at a time when the health care system in Botswana was not equipped to handle infertility and was just beginning to make treatment more available for HIV/AIDS. Nikki's and Sophia's stories thus illustrate how life is managed when living with infertility and HIV/AIDS. Their accounts were given during a time when anti-retrovirals (ARVs) were not yet freely available in the country, and the options for HIV/AIDS care were extremely limited. Their travels abroad were a crucial step in managing infertility, and possibly into successful conception while being HIV positive. Their accounts give evidence of a shift from an understanding of infertility that highlights the social aspects of this condition to a somatic understanding of infertility – the latter becoming more important in the following generation.

Making Bodies that Procreate: A Second Generation of Educated Professionals and ARTs

The second generation of women in my study had benefited from the country's rapid economic growth. In their thirties at the time of interview, it was common for these women to have travelled to Johannesburg, London, or any other place in the world. The two women, Maria and Lorato, whose stories I introduce here, had both enjoyed university education and had spent some time in the UK for studies or work. They were both financially well off, one working in finance and the other being an entrepreneur involved in various businesses (most recently in media).

I interviewed seventeen women in this generation. Their accounts of their reproductive histories were noticeably more biomedically exact and accurate concerning their clinical condition and, in general, my conversations with them were much more body-centred than those I had had with the older generation. The body-centeredness of their talk might partly be attributed to the fact that, because we were of a similar age, they felt more confident talking with me about matters of the body, while older women might have felt more awkward in communicating their condition to a younger and unmarried woman. These younger women had grown up in a society marked by HIV/AIDS. Since their teenage years, they had been exposed to education about health and sexuality through HIV prevention campaigns and in school; these campaigns tend to highlight the physical aspects of reproduction. Significantly, for this group the internet had provided a source of knowledge and communication that they had used in order to inform themselves not only about issues of fertility, but about discourses on health and the body in general. In addition to the internet, glossy magazines available for sale in Gaborone's fanciest shopping mall not only tell people what to eat and how to spend their leisure time but also 'educate' them on all matters concerning how to keep themselves fit and healthy. Weekly columns, such as Dr Kiran Bhagad's health consultancy in the weekly newspaper *The Voice*, inform people in Gaborone about general health problems and contribute to a popular and biomedically based knowledge and awareness of the body and health. Educated professionals are therefore part of a global trend of health-centeredness, in which physical well-being, the functioning body and its manipulation are highlighted. This knowledge influences how they care for their bodies in everyday life. Maria for instance, talked quite extensively about body weight and her concerns about gaining too much weight, which explains her regular visits to a fitness centre. Controlling and manipulating body weight and appearance was seen as crucial for maintaining a sense of femininity.

Maria and Lorato both conceived using IVF. Having well-paid positions and husbands in well-paid jobs, Maria and Lorato were only able to pursue the course they did because they could afford a cost-intensive fertility programme. The total cost of this treatment for Lorato and her husband, including travel and examinations, was about 100,000 BWP (around 7,800 GBP). In contrast, many other 'second generation' women I talked to could not afford the high costs of IVF and, like Sophia, hoped to get a loan or support from their parents. A significant level of affluence was therefore a precondition for Maria's and Lorato's access to ART, and reflects the stratification of reproduction in terms of income, as mentioned above.

Lorato and Maria, both aged 34 when I interviewed them, had discovered their fertility problem early on in their reproductive histories. At the age of 26 Maria had been trying for two years to become pregnant. During this time, she had visited a gynaecologist who worked at the Gaborone Private Hospital. He examined her and her husband, and did not find any physical cause for her infertility. Being an advocate of natural conception, he advised her to be patient and wait and see. She followed his advice and in fact became pregnant within two years. The pregnancy, however, turned out to be ectopic, and she described losing not only the foetus but also one of her fallopian tubes. During that time, she was desperate and her anxiety grew. Left with only one fallopian tube, she worried that her chances of a pregnancy had diminished. In addition, she feared that she might have another ectopic pregnancy and lose the other tube too. She changed to a female gynaecologist, the same one that Lorato consulted. When she changed doctors she had already familiarised herself with the medical problem of 'infertility' on the internet and in chat forums. Not wanting to lose any more time, she decided to seek the help of a specialist clinic in South Africa and enrolled in an IVF programme. After two years and three IVF cycles she became pregnant and, when I visited her at home in Gaborone, she had just given birth to her second child, again with the help of IVF (interview in Gaborone, 14 October 2011).

Lorato had a similar story to tell. She had experienced menstrual irregularities since the onset of her menarche. At 26, shortly after her marriage, and following three years working in the UK, Maria decided to have children, but she feared that she might encounter fertility problems. Her gynaecologists confirmed her suspicion and put her on Clomid treatment after doing the necessary examinations and tests. After three months, she had still not become pregnant. Her gynaecologists continued the treatment, however she became impatient as she was not satisfied with the treatment she was receiving; she went onto the internet and informed herself about 'infertility'. There, she not only learned that Clomid treatment should not be given for longer than three months but also about the possibilities of IVF. She went back to the gynaecologist and confronted her with her newly acquired knowledge. Like Maria, she decided to go through IVF, and she conceived after two cycles (interview in Gaborone, 10 October 2011).

Maria was a strong advocate of controlled conception. Despite her family's and friends' gentle admonition to be patient, she insisted on getting IVF treatment. And, she said, in her case there were so many things that they discovered during the treatment that it was really worth it. They found, for instance, that her vagina was too acidic and thus hindered the movement of her husband's sperm into the womb. 'If I had just sat back and waited,' she stated, 'they would never have found out and I would have lost time'. She also talked about her anxiety and setbacks during the treatment, such as a miscarriage after the second round of IVF. When she finally succeeded in becoming pregnant, she insisted on having a Caesarean section even though doctors, relatives and friends told her that a natural birth was healthier: 'After all I have been through, I didn't want anything to go wrong again', she said. Maria was a woman who insisted on retaining control of her reproductive agency, even against the advice of her gynaecologist, her mother, and her friends. Those who advised her 'to take it easy' and 'to relax', Maria dismissed, citing medical reasons derived from her new-found knowledge. This generation's narratives do not highlight the pressure and sometimes violence that feature in the older women's accounts. They appear far more independent and self-determined in their reproductive decisions. This includes an autonomy vis-à-vis their gynaecologists as well as vis-à-vis their natal families.

Lorato and Maria are examples of women of this generation who are becoming increasingly knowledgeable about the biological processes that shape and define their bodies and who use biomedical technologies in order to fulfil their reproductive wishes. This was in contrast with the older generation interviewed, whose bodies were not a ready subject of conversation. The younger women appeared to insist on doing everything possible in order to 'repair' a body that seemed to fail them in their reproductive desires. The younger generation adhere to an idea of fertility that can be produced by reproductive technologies, and uphold a biomedically informed view of health.

ART and Agency in the Context of HIV/AIDS

In their quest for conception and the modes through which they were able to fulfil their desires, educated professionals' biographies, drawn from two different generations, reflect a form of 'stratified reproduction' (Colen 1995). Albeit in different ways, both generations were able to access possibilities for fertility treatment that were unavailable to those who lacked sufficient financial resources and possibilities for overseas travel. While the younger generation appeared to be advocates of the paradigm of the 'make-ability' of life (Franklin 1995), women in the older generation were faced with little knowledge and few facilities concerning infertility (as well as concerning HIV/AIDS). Thus, being young, educated and wealthy contributed to women's ability to shape their reproductive lives according to their wishes. Lorato and Maria might be thought of as joining a global trend in which belief is placed in the growing importance of biological aspects of fertility and health, and the potential of biomedical technologies to overcome the body's failings. In Botswana, these are reinforced by the presence of the HIV virus that has enhanced biomedical care as well as biomedical knowledge of the body. Their story also speaks of a diversification of health care and knowledge; their HIV status never played a role in their interviews.

From my interview material, it is hard to judge where, as argued by Franklin, agency turns into constraint. The two younger women in this study had both insisted on their right to choose their own way of conceiving, even against the recommendation of their gynaecologists and families. Women of the older generation did not suggest that IVF or hormonal treatments were done under social pressure. Nikki and Sophia showed that their lives were marked by many social, economic and cultural constraints and pressures, including turbulent marriages, jealous and violent husbands and HIV/AIDS. Remarkably, in this generation, educated professionals experience similar constraints and pressures irrespective of their original social background. Analysing their accounts suggests that their quest for conception was overshadowed by traumatic experiences in their marriages, of which their childlessness appears as but one saddening aspect. Having grown up in a medical system that lacked facilities and knowledge, they seemed to accept that medical aid could not help much with their desire for children. For them fertility care in the US and UK represented a new possibility to cope with infertility and possibly also with an HIV infection.

From a critical perspective, one might argue that these technologies subject women to painstaking and cost intensive procedures with only moderate success rates, especially if they have passed their prime fertile years. Arguing from the point of view of those I interviewed, ARTs represent a tool of empowerment. The narratives of the second generation stress the moments of self-governance via the control of their reproductive bodies and health, and without references to their HIV status. In that way, the story of this second generation is also a story of hope. It allows insights into a society in which at least some privileged few have instruments and means to empower themselves against the pressure of family, friends and husbands, and irrespective of their HIV status.

Acknowledgements

This research was possible only with the support of the Fritz Thyssen Foundation and the Max Planck Institute for Social Anthropology, Halle. It was conducted with the permission of the Ministry of Labour and Home Affairs as well as the Ministry of Health, of the Gaborone Private Hospital (Dr Music and Dr Eaton) and Bokamoso Private Hospital (Dr Abebe). I thank all the institutions and people involved who have supported my research. My special thanks go to Abigail Morgan (Women's Health Nurse at Bokamoso) and Pastor Seithamo, who actively helped me make contact with patients and church members. Pearl Sechele and Abigile and John Hamathi have assisted me during my research. I thank especially John Hamathi for inspiring conversations and his help in connecting me with the right people as well as Dr Sethunya Mosime, Professor Godisan Mokoodi and Professor Treasa Galvin from the Department of Social Science, and Professor Musa Dube and Professor Francis Nkomasana from Theology and Religious Studies at the University of Botswana. Last but not least I want to thank Professor Rijk van Dijk from the ASC, Leiden, who introduced me to these colleagues.

Notes

1. This finding refers to a series of interviews I conducted with educated professionals who were aged between sixty and eighty. One example, of a head teacher, may demonstrate my point. The eighty-year-old woman had been to training college in Lesotho in the 1930s, after which she returned back to Botswana, got married at the age of 21 and started working. She delivered her first child at the age of 23, and her third and last child at the age of 28. Unlike her peers and siblings who had children when they were aged sixteen to eighteen, she postponed child birth in order to receive her professional training. Later, it was important to her to be able to manage a job as well as child raising and therefore used contraceptives throughout her marriage to prevent any further pregnancies (interview in Gaborone, 13 November 2011).
2. Hysterosalpingography (HSG) is a radiologic procedure to investigate the shape of the uterine cavity and the fallopian tubes.
3. In order to ensure the anonymity of my interviewees I changed all their names, and disguised other identity markers such as regional belonging and professions.
4. Clomid is a common hormonal treatment to support ovulation. In many places in Africa it is often the only treatment available for women who wish to conceive.
5. She told me about his HIV status when she talked about her husband's life *after* their marriage. It remains unclear whether he was positive already during their marriage.

Astrid Bochow is a Research Fellow at the Max Plank Institute for Social Anthropology. She is interested in reproduction, kinship, Pentecostalism, youth (age), and medical anthropology, and has conducted fieldwork in Botswana (Garbarone in the South East District) and Ghana (Kumasi in the Ashanti Region, and Accra and Endwa in the Greater Accra Region).

Chapter 8

A Child Cannot Be Bought?

Economies of Hope and Failure when Using ARTs in Mali

Viola Hörbst

Ah, a child cannot be bought
Mrs Kona, a child cannot be bought,
In fact a child is in the hand of Allah
Dear mamas a child cannot be bought my God
If you could have a child with gold
I would give it to you
Your father owns the gold of Buré
Mrs Kona, a child cannot be bought
If you could buy a child with cows
I would find them for you

From the song '*Dinkole*' (Issue of Children)
By the Malian singer Nainy Diabaté

Mali, the country in focus in this chapter, covers mostly desert or semi-desert regions and is ranked among the poorest countries in the world. The Malian population is nearly 16 million (WPR 2014). The capital, Bamako, had about 1 million inhabitants in 1998, 1.7 million in 2006 and 2 million by 2010. Its annual urban growth rate is the highest in Africa and ranks sixth in the world (Philippe 2009). Population growth remains high at 3 per cent, and the total fertility rate is still around 6.4 children per woman (WPR 2014). Maternal mortality is estimated to be nearly 6 per 1,000 births (WHO 2014), infant mortality is 1 death per 10 live births (WPR 2014) and 128 children out of 1,000 die before the age of 5 (WHO 2014). The gross domestic product amounts to around 7.7 billion euros, equating to 485 euros per capita (World Bank 2014).

These numbers reinforce the commonly held image of poverty reigning Mali. Yet, at the same time you may find yourself in the rush hour trapped between many huge limousines. In the newer districts of Bamako, extravagant villas of different size, style and form, line up side by side. Weddings are significant occasions for a lavish show of wealth. One might wonder how it is that one of the poorest countries in the world has such a visibly emergent 'middle class' and affluence. One begins to question the formal statistics and the nature of informal markets, which are definitely not limited to selling peanuts and mangos in the streets but also cover a huge range of activities, including the production of textiles and selling cars and pharmaceuticals.

But bridging the enormous ethnic, religious and economic diversity visible among the 16 million Malians is the great importance attached to having children. As has been reported from across sub-Saharan Africa, children are highly valued because they deliver additional working hands to families; they provide economic as well as physical support in old age; and they ensure the continuity of the lineage and the family's connection with ancestral spirits (Kielman 1998; Gerrits 2002; Leonard 2002). To produce children is a major objective for married couples and is equated with being recognised as a fully fledged adult. For Malian women who are living within extended families, with co-wives and frequently demanding sisters- and mothers-in-law, children are often the only people they can totally rely on (Hörbst 2012). Children grant women an occupation in daily life, as well as some security and comfort in marriage when love and passion decreases and/or a second wife moves in. Children thus enable women to have some emotional and economic independence from their husbands, and are key when it comes to respect from the extended family. Since having children is a prime social requirement, childless couples go to enormous lengths to become parents.

There are several options that couples may pursue when coming to terms with involuntary childlessness. Besides 'social solutions' (fostering children, extramarital cohabitation), many Malians resort to religious interventions (animistic, Islamic and Christian prayers and rituals), and so-called 'traditional' methods (for example, herbal decoctions). Moreover, private and public gynaecological clinics provide classic biomedical treatment (such as hormone cocktails, endoscopic dilatation, and hormonal stimulation). In the last few years some clinics have begun to offer highly sophisticated ARTs, including intrauterine insemination, IVF and ICSI. ARTs performed both outside and inside Mali are becoming an attractive option for Malian women and men who are involuntarily childless. These bio-techniques provide important advantages compared to traditional solutions for childless couples, fostering the hope that they will be able to have their own genetic offspring. Successful treatment with ARTs allows women to become visibly pregnant, which is crucial in countering the stigmatisation of childlessness (Hörbst 2012). However, despite being substantially less costly than in Europe or the United States, such treatments remain accessible only for a tiny minority in Mali.

As ARTs travel from Europe to Africa, they bring into relation a variety of actors, institutions and technologies. I have highlighted elsewhere how these relations operate on different scales within global ART medicoscapes operating in Bamako (Hörbst 2012). In this chapter, I will focus particularly on women, the local end users of ARTs, in order to show the ways in which using ARTs in Bamako embeds them in transnational therapeutic networks. Like Charris Cussins (1996), I use the notion of 'doing' ARTs to emphasise Bamakonian women's objectification when undergoing ARTs and how this also forms part of their agency when it comes to achieving the ultimate aim of having a child. By describing the changes over time when women prepare for, undergo and evaluate interactions with ARTs in Bamako, I want to link their moves to the socio-material contexts in which their lives are embedded in order to carve out how economies of hope and failure speak to specifically Bamakonian contexts regarding social order and everyday life. Drawing on data from my repeated fieldwork stays in Mali (2004–2012) I will present several women's 'ART stories', each of which shows distinct constraints in their ways of navigating infertility. These case studies are arranged in two blocks: the first centres on women's trajectories at the beginning of their treatment processes and the second on changes in tactics when treatments fail repeatedly.

Starting to Use ARTs in Bamako

Djeneba and Seydou

I met Djeneba in 2006 while observing consultations in a gynaecological clinic in Bamako. Born in 1979, Djeneba is a lively woman who works for an international NGO. In 2002, she married Seydou, who is eight years older than her and is employed at the customs authority. To talk with me, Djeneba drove me in her Mercedes limousine to their house in the rapidly growing outskirts of Bamako. Members of both their extended families visit them regularly, although they live in various villas scattered around Bamako. Djeneba's newly built villa stretches over two floors and includes garages for the couple's two cars. The vast living room mirrors the couple's prosperity in the form of Western-style lounges, and armchairs in white imitation leather. Several air conditioners complete the impression, as do the huge widescreen television and video recorder dominating the room.

Sitting on her couch in 2006, Djeneba started to tell me her story. When, six months after the wedding, she had still not conceived, they visited the university clinic in Bamako to find out if anything was wrong. While she had minor problems with a uterine tumour (myoma), her husband was diagnosed with a very low sperm count (oligospermia). A relative, who was trained as medical doctor, gave Djeneba the address of an infertility clinic in Morocco, which she contacted. What they asked was only for the necessary pre-analysis and the remunerations for the specialists; but, excluding the costs of the flights, accommodation, and the transport between airport and clinic, that still accounted for nearly 5,000 euros.

While clinics in Togo, Benin and France were also under discussion, they finally found out about a private clinic in Bamako, where insemination and IVF were offered. Djeneba and Seydou went there, in order to save money on otherwise expensive flights and accommodation. Moreover, using ARTs locally would allow them to continue their professional and daily lives and provide additional emotional comfort. Seydou was treated again with hormones. After six months the number as well as the vitality of Seydou's sperm increased and the doctor suggested trying insemination. On the first attempt, Djeneba conceived, and in spring 2007 her child was born. Sadly, the baby died after one week due to an occlusion of the oesophagus that was treated too late.

At the beginning, Djeneba and Seydou approached the financing of their treatments in a cooperative way. With two incomes (one from an international NGO that pays comparatively high salaries, and one from the customs authority where informal incidental earnings are said to be common) this expenditure was quite feasible. Additionally, Djeneba participated in *tontines*: popular saving associations in West Africa mainly enacted among women at all economic levels. A *tontine* commonly gathers around eight to twenty women, who each contribute a monthly amount from one euro up to three hundred euros, or even more. Each month the members hold a social meeting and the sum gathered by all the women is handed over to one of the participants.

Within their relationship, Seydou acknowledged that his male-factor hypofertility diagnosis was the reason for their childlessness. However, Seydou informed no one in his family about his condition, and Djeneba also concealed the information: 'In most cases of infertility, people here say it comes from the women. Of course people are aware that in principle it could also come due to problems of the husband. But [because of] the way in which he had supported me, I did not want to expose him to that disgrace and shame'.

For many years, Djeneba thus shouldered the provocations and negative comments about her childlessness uttered particularly by her mother-in-law and sisters-in-law, all of whom assumed that she was the cause of the ongoing 'problem'. Djeneba told me that after the birth and death of their baby these insulting comments lessened. However, 'it is not yet over,' she continued, 'but now they all pray for me'.

While Djeneba and Seydou's information about the variants of ARTs came principally from friends, some of whom are clinical practitioners, and also from the gynaecological experts they have consulted, this was not the case for Kadidja, another Bamakonian woman who used ARTs locally in Bamako.

Kadidja and Abdou

Kadidja, born in 1975, grew up in Mali and then studied computer science in France. Since 2002, she has been employed by a bank in Bamako. In 2003 she married Abdou, who also works in finance. They live together in one of the old and popular quarters of Bamako's city centre, within the compound of Abdou's family. This special type of compound encloses a winding concrete house with three floors as well as a couple of further mud buildings on the ground floor. Kadidja and Abdou occupy a three-room apartment on the second floor, which has an air conditioner in the living room as well as a television and Western-style sofas. The room is, however, less spacious, elegant and luxurious than the equivalent in Djeneba's house.

In contrast to Djeneba, Kadidja was not informed in the first instance by doctors about advanced technological options. Instead, she herself accessed the websites of several French clinics, but then she also started treatment in Bamako. After a first miscarriage in 2005, Kadidja and her husband travelled to France to repeat the analysis. There the doctors told her that her right tube was slightly adhered, but this, they explained, was not problematic. Examining her husband, the doctors found a low sperm count and suggested an IUI (intra-uterine insemination). Kadidja and Abdou did their first IUI in France, but unfortunately without success. When they returned to Bamako, Kadidja made two further attempts with IUI, and in 2007 she finally gave birth to a healthy child.

Unlike Djeneba and many other Malian women, Kadidja claimed not to feel any social pressure from her in-laws. According to Kadidja, they are 'very religious' and understanding; another reason for the absence of pressure is that they are not the only couple in the family that does not have children yet. Similarly, Kadidja said she did not feel pressurised by work colleagues, who would regularly inform her about acquaintances who had successfully undergone various procedures. While her mother and sister also pushed her towards treatments, Kadidja interpreted this behaviour as a gesture intended to help rather than to pressure her: 'I think these are people who are worried about me … I understand, they do it for me, in favour with me, therefore it doesn't stress me'.

A close friend, who is also involuntarily childless in her marriage, helps Kadidja to navigate these dense social situations positively, as she explained: 'It's very good to have a friend who is in the same situation. Well, I cannot imagine how to speak more openly about all this because, with others, I do not know, I feel embarrassed'.

Since their situation is shared, Kadidja can find emotional consolation through this relationship. Although Abdou's physical condition is diagnosed as the major reason for their infertility, the initiative to use ARTs came from Kadidja. As in the case of Djeneba and her husband Seydou, Abdou has not informed his family about his infertility. Kadidja is similarly discrete but has told her mother and her younger sister. While both partners are in well-paid employment, the treatment is still expensive for them, although not prohibitively so. This is in contrast to the case of Salifa, below, for whom money for ARTs and a cooperative partner were both lacking.

Salifa

Salifa, born in 1964, lives with her second husband in a conventional compound belonging to his family. Their compound is in an older, popular quarter of the city and is a rather typical example of this still very common form of housing in Bamako. Around central rectangular patios, which often have shady trees, are low buildings made of mud or concrete. They are divided into separate one or two room areas with doors opening to the patio. On the patio the cooking and the laundry are done and children play while the compound's inhabitants meet and chat or take their meals. Typically, a compound comprises the (male) head of the family, his wives(s) and children, several of his brothers with their wives and children, widowed or divorced sisters with children, and his parents. In her compound, Salifa and her husband have a living room and a bedroom at their disposal. The living room is equipped with some rather worn out sofas, shelf units with souvenirs, photos and porcelain, and an old television. Salifa was trained in accounting and worked for many years in a pharmaceutical enterprise. When I first met her in 2004, she was unemployed but spent her time engaged in the informal sale of fabrics.

In 1991 Salifa married her first husband. The marriage lasted for eight years, without her getting pregnant. Her husband was diagnosed as having severe oligospermia, and in the end she filed a petition for divorce despite the opposition of her husband and in-laws. In 1998 she married her second husband, whose wife had died young. She cares for his two sons from his first marriage as well as for a foster child, given to her by her second husband's younger brother, whose wife died during birthing. The years have passed, but her second marriage also remains childless, although various gynaecologists have been unable to find any physical cause. Her husband was not willing to undergo any analyses, arguing that he had previously produced two children. He also refused to finance any medical treatments concerning their childlessness.

Salifa feels accepted by her in-laws in the compound. Her mother-in-law, the eldest and, in social terms, highest-ranking woman living there, had also experienced childlessness. Thus, no one in the compound dares to bother Salifa with sneering remarks about her childlessness, because such a comment would be considered a rude offence against her mother-in-law. However, Salifa worries about her increasing age and about her husband's intention to take a second wife. Owing to her unemployment, Salifa was bound to daily life in the compound and became increasingly uneasy with her thoughts circling around her childlessness and what – in her perception – equated to a useless existence.

Salifa had already heard about ARTs via television and would undertake such a treatment without hesitation. Two brothers suggested that Salifa should go to Paris, where they live, in order to use ART there. Her brother-in-law, the father of her foster child, would have also contributed to such an intervention – but Salifa was denied a visa for France. She herself could not afford to undertake such a treatment in Mali or Senegal. Her brothers and brother-in-law dismissed such an option because they doubted the likelihood of success, especially since her husband was uncooperative. Although Salifa herself apparently had no fertility problems, she lacked the basic cooperation of her husband and therefore dismissed the possibility of using ART. When I met her again in 2010, she had found work in a canteen, allowing her to earn some additional money. Disenchanted and tearful, Salifa told me that she had stopped all treatments and was trying not to think any more about having a child.

Mariam

Like Salifa, Mariam is also over forty – but she is preparing for ARTs. Her husband, Brahmina, unlike Salifa's, does not actively try to prevent Mariam from seeking treatment, and Mariam's overall situation is also rather different. Born in 1966, she is a trained nurse and employed in a public hospital. In 1997 she became the second wife of Brahmina, a successful businessman. Brahmina already has three children with his first wife, while his marriage with Mariam has so far remained childless. Mariam lives with a foster child in a small house situated in a popular quarter of Bamako's suburbs. Her husband visits her for two days and nights at a time, alternating between his two wives. Although Mariam has a reasonable income, her financial and living situation certainly does not compare with those of Kadidja or Djeneba. When I met her, at the end of 2007, she had been diagnosed with premature ageing of the ovaries, and was planning IVF in Bamako using donor ova. She explained that her husband was not going to contribute financially: 'Brahmina already has children with his first wife; therefore he prefers to invest his money in his house rather than in such an expensive treatment for me. For him this is not so important. The second wife herself has to look how to manage this'.

Although she is disappointed, Mariam organises the money. She saves part of her monthly salary in her bank account and also invests around 100 euros per month in six *tontines*, which gives her a pay-off of nearly 700 euros every 10 months, and 600 every 20 months. In addition, she informally sells food products at the clinic. While Mariam conceals the treatments from her husband's family, her sisters are informed about her activities and give her emotional as well as financial support. Her elder sister, who lives permanently in France, helps her with the cost of drugs, and also sends extra money from time to time.

Discussion of the Case Studies

As the four ARTs stories reveal, social and financial circumstances, combined the support women may (or may not) receive from friends, family, husbands and in-laws, determine their ability to use ARTs. The four women presented were each considering pursuing ART outside of Mali, but in the end preferred to undergo treatment at home, for financial reasons and for what might be thought of as emotional benefits. Women pursued various strategies to accumulate the resources needed to undertake ARTs. Formal-sector employment was often a crucial element of this, along with access to official saving options and small credit lines. Informal incomes and saving options, such as *tontines*, are important supplements. Mariam, Kadidja and Djeneba had both formal and informal options at their disposal, while Salifa had to get by with only *tontines* and income from cloth trading. Yet Salifa had affluent brothers, who were willing to pay for her treatment. Having access to extended family networks, especially those living abroad and/or who are relatively well-off, provides an alternative when the husband is not willing or able to pay.

However, even if husbands did not contribute financially, some minimum level of cooperation was crucial for accessing ART treatment and for a basic willingness to accept male-factor infertility as a reason – both aspects were lacking in Salifa's case. In the case of Kadidja's and Djeneba's husbands, neither had any children of their own and both were prepared to accept their diagnoses (although not publicly, and with varying degrees of acceptance). But in Salifa's case, even though biomedical diagnosis indicated that her husband was probably the one 'responsible' for their marital childlessness, the fact that he had procreated with his previous spouse allowed him to effectively ignore these hints and deny any moral or financial support to Salifa. His lack of cooperation effectively precluded Salifa from taking the opportunities offered by her brothers to go ahead with ARTs. It is therefore not simply the husband's financial situation that is important in women's access to ARTs, but the husband's *cooperation* in pursuing treatment options – or, at least, a basic willingness to undergo diagnosis with the concomitant risk of discovering his own biological shortcoming. While Mariam's husband already had children, he did not refuse to cooperate with his wife, even though he did not provide much in the way of financial support.

Women's access to ART is thus dependent on the degree to which the husband is willing to accept his diagnosis, and whether there are children from earlier or parallel marriages that might relieve the social pressure on him. Although finances are an overarching theme for all women, and concern them far more than worries about physical risks or possible treatment failure, the financial position of the individuals/couple alone is not the whole story. The opportunity for treatment is often also dependent on affluent relatives who can contribute and organise financial support. These financial options particularly form an important part when ART treatments have to be repeated. But how do strategies, discourses and evaluations of women change when constant failure comes to the fore? And which topics become central issues of concern for the women when treatments are repeated and fail again? In the next section I will follow these questions and describe the ways in which women deal with (repeated) failure when using ART in Bamako.

Continuing to Use ARTs: Secrecies, Failures and Worries

In the early stages of ART treatments, women's worries about the nature of procedures they would undergo or the risks they would face were usually not expressed. Some women spoke about the failure of earlier treatments and the pains they had experienced but, in all cases, the hope to have a child was paramount, and this overshadowed concerns about the risks associated with these biotechnical procedures.

Kadidja and Abdou

Neither Kadidja nor Abdou informed their families about the real nature of their fertility treatment. Even Kadidja's mother and sister did not know any details. However, the interventions did not bother Kadidja:

> It is only a bit tiring to do all these treatments and afterwards there is no result – this is demotivating, discouraging. In the beginning I was not worried about that, it did not stress me. Well, now, I start to ask myself 'will this work?' ... For the moment, I calm myself; I tell myself there is no reason why it should not work. Even the last time I told my husband this. He asked me whether we will ever have children, I told him no, we will have some! The problem is the money, I want to say; if the IUI is not working, I have my ova, you have your sperm; then we will make immediately an IVF – no problem.

During the hormonal treatment of Kadidja's husband, his sperm quality increased significantly, a result both were happy about. Yet, at the beginning of 2006, she had a serious quarrel with her husband, as she explains:

> It was about the reason. The doctor asked him to do a treatment and he did not want to. Abdou told me that there is no problem with him; the doctor has studied the structure of his sperm, well, he said, there is no serious problem. I told him, 'OK, but there is still a decrease in mobility and a decrease in quantity of sperm, no?' Abdou said, 'Yes, but I don't have a problem'. Then I got angry, we quarrelled very heavily. Afterwards I calmed down. ... We discussed and I told him, if there are treatments to make then he must do it. He resumed the treatments and we started again.

Finally, Kadidja's husband continued to cooperate smoothly. But, through the increase of processing time and repeated failures, Kadidja's confidence diminished. While she comforted herself that IUI is not yet the treatment of last resort, she was beginning to worry about how to shoulder the higher costs if IVF was to be needed.

Mariam

In 2009, Mariam had completed 'her project', that is, an IVF cycle with donor ova. For her husband, aiming for a child with Mariam by using ART was clearly not his priority. Although he is not against using ARTs he does not support her either financially or morally. He did not usually accompany her to the treatments, he did not care for her in the clinic after transfer, and he did not fetch her home afterwards.

While Mariam informed Brahmina about the different steps of the IVF procedure, she did not tell him that donor ova were being used, as she was afraid he would not agree. She did not appear to feel bad about omitting this detail, but rather used this tactical step to protect her 'project'. The doctor, although unhappy about it, was accepting. In Malian contexts, a couple is not necessarily seen as a unit in such treatments. The plan to use donor ova was only shared between the doctor, the embryologist, Mariam and her younger sister who would be the donor. Unfortunately, Mariam's sister's ova were not of sufficient quality. Therefore, IVF was done with the ova of Mariam's 19-year-old niece, which involved sharing the secret and thus increasing the risk of potential disclosure.

Everything started fine, with Mariam in a very positive mood. Seven ova were extracted and two days later two embryos were implanted in her uterus. As she stated: 'This, now, will be the end of my suffering – I had the child on my mind. When the doctor told me on the phone, "I am sorry, it did not work", I was totally down. I was at the edge, feeling very bad. I didn't want to talk with anyone; I didn't want to see anyone. I became ill and stayed in bed. I stayed away from work for another two weeks'.

All Mariam's savings had been spent on the IVF procedure and the pharmaceuticals needed. The doctor, she complained, had not informed her about his rates of success and failure, and she never received an explanation as to why the intervention failed. For months, Mariam did not want to see the gynaecologist. During our discussions, Mariam did not complain about the physical effects of the treatment, or the pain or risks for herself. Instead, what she worried about after the first IVF treatment was her niece, who gave her ova:

> 'I would prefer that my niece won't do it a second time. The epidural continued to have an effect for two days. She couldn't get up normally, that was quite traumatising for her. The girl won't say no, if I ask her again, but also I am worried about her fertility, I don't want to risk anything with her'.

She would prefer to use an anonymous donor, she continued. Using another relative would be possible but she would have to explain the situation and asking such a favour is not very pleasant. Moreover, this also would involve spreading the secret to other family members, so it would again increase the risk that her husband might learn about it. Despite failing to become pregnant, her sister encouraged her not to lose heart with the Malian doctor and to try it again there, as it was cheaper than travelling abroad. Finally, at the end of 2010, she carried out the IVF with ova from an anonymous donor in Bamako – but again it was in vain: 'All the money! Each time I have to pay 850,000 FCFA [roughly 1,300 euros]. Each time I have to find it myself as my husband doesn't participate. Only my sister and her husband in France are continuously helping me'.

It is not only the loss of such a large amount of money itself that troubles Mariam. It is also about the significant loss of money in a Bamakonian context where many people are in need and are entitled to ask family members whom they know to have money to lend small sums. As Mariam has repeatedly spent large amounts of money on IVF cycles, this puts her in socially problematic situations. She should lend money, but she is not in a position to do so and she cannot discuss why. This puts her into the stressful condition of constantly needing excuses when questions of money lending arise. This is doubly problematic given that childless women, according to mainstream Malian norms, are judged as being bad and jealous. One means for childless women to counter this stereotyping is to show particular generosity, giving presents to those around them. Having spent such large amounts of money while a lot of people (members of the *tontines*, for example) know that Mariam should have money left brings her into social difficulties.

Djeneba

In 2007, when she was doing the first insemination, Djeneba told me that she did not mind the treatment at all. She said that for her it is less painful than other treatments such as a hysterosalpingogram (that in Bamako seems to be done quite often without pain killers). Since then, Djeneba had had another three inseminations, all of which failed. In early 2009, the doctor requested another hysterosalpingogram and diagnosed that both her fallopian tubes were now blocked. Thus, he suggested trying IVF by using the couple's gametes. Djeneba and Seydou followed his recommendation at the end of 2009. Ten ova were extracted and 6 embryos were produced. While Djeneba never complained about the insemination procedure and all the injections she had to suffer, she experienced the hormonal stimulation for IVF rather differently:

> A staff member from the clinic came to my house; we arranged the price between us. He took 3.50 euro – that was very fair and ok. If

> I would have gone myself, I would have needed two taxis, one to go and one to return, that costs around 5 euro. Thus, I earned with this. But in general it was too much obligation, it needed too much time and it was too stressing. With IVF it was sometimes up to four injections a day. Imagine! After ten days I was tired of these treatments; I didn't even want to look at a syringe – and I would have loved to stop everything. But I continued, because of my target to have a child.

However, during these years Djeneba's husband remained a highly supportive companion; he contributed to the treatments, gave her deep moral support and comforted her in the face of repeated failure to conceive. Notwithstanding the social pressure put on him, he did not give in by taking a second wife in order to increase his chances of having children. For Djeneba, each failure of the treatment seemed to be more burdensome and was then topped with doing further IVF. The continuous failures and spiralling costs left her bitter and desperately disappointed. When the doctor suggested doing another IVF with donor ova due to the condition of her tubes and her increased age, Djeneba decided to stop: 'I have too many bad memories ... I don't want to become any longer traumatised. I think that I won't find my happiness, my chance with this doctor'.

Impacts of Failures when Using ARTs in Bamako

Worries about money accompany all women using ARTs in Bamako. In the beginning, the women's attitudes are focused on hope and shaped by confidence and a kind of pride that these high-tech solutions are provided in their African home country and not just in rich Western ones. However, financing ARTs is a constant worry for most women who resort to this avenue to become a parent. In cases of success, the money spent is forgotten; but in cases of failure, the women have to face deception and depression as well as the loss of their money. In Malian terms, the money to finance one round of IVF is a huge sum that could be invested more sustainably. Additionally, with each failing cycle, it becomes more difficult to keep the spirit focused on hope. Kadidja, for example, starts doubting her bodily condition, worrying that it might block her from achieving her goal via ARTs. Mariam is repeatedly questioning certain single steps of the treatment and contests the doctor's competence, as does Djeneba: 'Yes, I got it straight that there is no certainty. But it is the doctors, they have not enough experience. Perhaps they have good results with insemination and a good rate of chances, but not with IVF. With IVF they have too few cases anyhow. With four inseminations, one IVF and one child lost due to their negligence – that is enough'.

Further, the women complain about their doctors' professionalism when confronted with failures. No explanation is given for why the intervention failed, for example, and the doctors do not seem to care about their emotional situation. They particularly challenge the absence of explanations and the lack of social care from their doctors although they were long-term patients in his clinic. Both aspects decrease confidence in his professionalism and responsibility. Djeneba highlighted this point when I asked her if she had confronted the doctor regarding her blocked tubes, which she assumes to be connected to the treatments:

> What would I gain with doing so? He will bother me with medical explanations I won't understand – that it is due to this or that; he will say this and thus, but he will never acknowledge his share ... The doctors here in Mali are like that. They won't tell you that they have done something, because they think you will tell other people, then they will lose their clients – they think you spoil their business!

As ARTs are found only in the private health sector in Mali, where patients have to pay for treatments out of their own pocket, repeated failure challenges the rules of this biomedical contract, as Mariam complains: 'He did not reimburse me anything – this at least he could do if his intervention doesn't work. At least 50 per cent he could have returned to me'. As with Mariam, other women tend to equate the provision of these treatments with other service markets. If good service is not provided, there is an expectation that at least part of the money should be given back to the customer. Added to doubts about doctors' competence and skills, these factors accelerate disillusionment in the biomedical field as a serious business. This complex also reduces the once-seen advantage of lower costs in Bamako, as Mariam states: 'Maybe somewhere else, even so it might be more expensive, it might be better done there? Perhaps it will be carried out in a more skilled way then? Maybe my chances for success will be higher there?'

All the women I interviewed had thought about going abroad for treatment in the beginning, and Kadidja had indeed realised her first IUI outside Mali. Repeated unsuccessful local ARTs interventions reinforced these women's desires for transnational interventions. After repeated failure of ART interventions, women began to associate ARTs in Europe with higher standards, higher medical competence, skills and technical equipment, as well as greater experience. To pay higher prices for such treatment brings an assumption of a better quality of care, just as higher prices for goods are often taken as markers of better quality.

In 2010 Mariam contacted an ART clinic in Dakar, Senegal; at the same time she visited her sister in France and consulted a clinic there. Djeneba and her husband finally went to Brussels in 2011, where they stayed in the large comfortable house of Djeneba's former schoolmate living there. In summer 2012, Djeneba and Seydou became the happy parents of twins. Both Mariam and Djeneba were able to pursue their original plan to seek ART outside Mali, but this possibility is limited to the most affluent only.

Economies of Hope and Failure

Women using ARTs in Bamako are, above all, concerned with financial worries. Although they belong to the more affluent parts of Malian society, ART demands serious financial investments. As women's ART trajectories show, in order to find the money during the period of preparation, the overarching problems are to do with convincing husbands and winning their financial commitment, or at least their basic agreement. In this first period of treatment, the women show high confidence in the competence and technical equipment of the local ART providers, and focus on the hope of success. Within this economy of hope, they struggle hard to get the means together to realise ART, but, during this period, they do not critique the commercial side of treatments, which seems at the time to form but a small part of their project. When ART treatment results in having a baby, the involved financial hardships are quickly forgotten as a characteristic feature of an economy of success. But in an ongoing process of further treatments, this begins to shift.

If treatments fail and have to be repeated, hope becomes harder and harder to maintain. Doubts start to grow about the chances of getting successful ART treatment in Bamako. Repeated treatment failure amplifies these women's stress in the management of entangled family relations, money and secrecies. As became notable in the stories presented above, emotional, social and financial limits are touched, as well as the limits of confidence in local doctors' competence and sincerity. Having done several ART treatments without having a baby, women somehow feel deceived in their expectations and investments. Their whole ART project somehow becomes reduced to its commercial side, a characteristic of what I call the economy of failure. Constant failures generate feelings of having been exposed to unfair business. Due to these feelings and experiences Malian women not only ask for better information and transparency as well as better standards of care, but, as I have shown, the women demand that doctors apply a stricter interpretation of fair commercial conventions as expressed in the idea that they should reimburse at least a percentage of the price in case of treatment failure. Failure of biomedical treatments in neo-liberal health markets bring about traits of moral economies claiming for a change in business handling.

This demand connects to a characteristic feature of ART treatments all over the world – the high uncertainty of assisted reproductive services. ARTs have a success rate between 15 and 50 per cent – the latter rate being only achieved in the world's top clinics. This fact exhibits a very low certainty, indeed a high risk of failure, while, at the same time, these biomedical services are particularly expensive and also demand a high physical investment, particularly from the women. Certainly, these aspects are a problem of ART treatments all over the world, but one that becomes particularly acute in unsuccessful interventions. To ask high prices for assisted reproductive technology treatments, with no reimbursement in case of failure, produces a series of dilemmas in the biomedical commercialisation of ARTs.

In most localities in the world, unsuccessful ART treatments puts the financial burden of failure exclusively on the clients' shoulders (and in Mali, these are disproportionately the shoulders of women, as these case stories have shown), even though success rates are relatively low. This equates to an unbalanced contract between providers and clients, where controllability, risk taking and paying high prices are unequally shared between the parties involved.

These unbalanced issues become more visible in contexts where no insurance schemes, or national governmental funding is available for ARTs, and patients mainly have to pay for these treatments out of their own pockets. Such factors are particularly relevant in developing countries where the normative and social pressures to have children are very high and acceptance of adoption may be low. However, there are women's groups starting activities, for instance in Mali and in Uganda, to promote adoption as an acceptable practice and a solution to infertility. Additionally, in developing countries, where effective quality control mechanisms for doctors and effective complaint procedures for patients are often lacking, this inequity seems to be particularly tangible and unfair. Even if patient lobby groups existed around infertility treatment, the cultural tendency to keep such interventions secret might well prevent effective complaints, as they have prevented patient groups becoming powerful in other countries (for more details see Hörbst and Wolf 2014).

The request made by Mariam and other Malian women to get a percentage of money reimbursed in case of failing ART interventions accentuate these configurations in which the extremely high uncertainty of assisted reproductive business is taking place: an uncertainty that rather turns treatments for women and couples into an exercise of 'betting on fate' as a European embryologist I spoke with in the field put it. The women's agency when using ART is not caught up in objectification in the clinic, but rather in the particular 'commercial traditions' ruling biomedical health systems.

However, these structural inequities are part of complex socio-cultural, historical and political configurations, taking place within (private) health markets acting untamed under neo-liberal banners, particularly in developing countries. To analyse this commercialisation from the point of failure opens a window not only to better understand the constraints of ART treatments in a more contextualised and nuanced way, but also highlights the way that biomedical services may be in tension with other conventions around doing business and having recourse in the event of dissatisfaction.

While money may not be able to buy a child directly, as the song of Nainy Diabaté cited at the beginning of the chapter suggests, high resources of 'gold', 'cows' or money definitely increase one's chances of obtaining a child through ARTs. Thus the consoling tone of Diabaté's words may leave a bitter aftertaste for poor women in Bamako who have no access to ARTs at all, and for women who undertake ARTs but with constant failure.

Acknowledgements

I would like to warmly thank Kate Hampshire and Bob Simpson for inviting me to contribute a chapter to this edited volume, as well as for their inspiring comments and recommendations on an earlier version. I also profited from anonymous reviewers' remarks for which I am grateful as well. The field research in 2004 and 2005 was financed by a scholarship from the women's representative at the Ludwig-Maximilian University of Munich within the framework of the University and Science Program, and was completed by a donation from the Friends of the Ludwig-Maximilian University of Munich. The research from 2006 to 2008 was financed by the German Research Foundation (DFG). Further field stays between 2009 and 2011 were sponsored by the Portuguese Foundation for Science and Technology (FCT). I am most grateful to these institutions. Above all I am most indebted to all women, men, institutions and practitioners with whom I worked during my research in Bamako. With respect for their privacy, personal names in this chapter have been changed.

Viola Hörbst (MA, PhD) is currently a freelance researcher, specialising in the anthropology of health. In her PhD thesis (1998–2002) she explored healing landscapes in rural Western Mexico, but in subsequent years has focused on infertility and ARTs in West Africa, mainly in Mali but also in Togo and Senegal (2004–2011). She recently headed a research group (2011–2013) investigating appropriations of ART practices in different sub-Saharan countries (Ghana, Mozambique, South Africa and Uganda). Her recent publications address issues of ARTs, transnational networks and technology transfer in sub-Saharan Africa.

Chapter 9

Practitioner Perspective

A View from Sri Lanka

Thilina S. Palihawadana and H.R. Seneviratne

As practitioners with experience of infertility and its treatment in Sri Lanka, we welcome the inclusion of chapters that focus explicitly on the growth and development of ARTs in resource-poor settings. In this commentary, we provide an illustrative case study from Sri Lanka, where both authors have experience practising and teaching reproductive medicine, and where ARTs have now been in place for nearly two decades. In our account, we present five key themes that resonate with the development of ARTs in the different country settings described in this part of the book. These themes are: endorsement of ARTs, access to ARTs, knowledge transfer, regulatory lag, and the complex integration of ARTs with other systems of belief and practice.

Sri Lanka: A Case in Point

Sri Lanka is a lower-middle income developing country in South Asia with a gross domestic income per capita of US$1,780. The health needs of the population are mainly met by the state sector national health service, which is non fee-levying. A private health sector is also available where the patients bear the total cost of treatment received. Health insurance is not widely accepted, although a small minority enjoy such benefits usually provided by the private sector. The provision of the service in the government health sector is through the Ministry of Health (MOH) while the regulation is by the Sri Lanka Medical Council. The MOH now has a unit managed by a deputy director general to monitor the services provided by private institutions. Postgraduate medical education is governed by the Postgraduate Institute of Medicine (PGIM) of the University of Colombo. The professional colleges, such as the Sri Lankan College of Obstetricians and Gynaecologists, play an advisory role to the PGIM and the Ministry of Health on the needs of the country within the speciality.

The true prevalence of infertility in the country is yet to be established. Many authorities believe it to be close to the universally accepted figure of 15 per cent worldwide, although the prevalence in many developing countries has been shown to be higher than this (Rutstein and Iqbal 2004). Infertility treatment has been provided in Sri Lanka in the state health sector as a part of general obstetrics and gynaecology, while advanced infertility services such as Assisted Reproductive Technologies (ARTs) are provided only by a few centres in the private sector. These private enterprises operate on a fee-levying basis. Such IVF centres have been in operation since the late 1990s but were staffed by visiting experts from overseas. Since the first IVF baby by the efforts of a complete Sri Lankan team was born in 2002, ART services within the country have developed and public awareness of this facility has increased. Alternative modalities of treatment such as indigenous medicines as well as religious and cultural ritual practices coexist in Sri Lanka. Some patients tend to follow these either in isolation or in combination with medical treatment, although they are advised to avoid combination therapy.

The Sri Lankan Experience of Infertility Care

The importance of infertility care has been well recognised in the country. From its inception in 1953, the Family Planning Association of Sri Lanka (FPA-SL) adopted both contraception and infertility services as its recognised goals (Chinnatamby 1970, 1990). The need for more advanced infertility treatment modalities within the country has also been recognised more recently by the Sri Lanka College of Obstetricians and Gynaecologists (SLCOG) and recommendations have been made to the Ministry of Health and the Postgraduate Institute of Medicine (PGIM) to train sub-specialists in the management of infertility.

Infertility treatment is one branch of medicine that has advanced rapidly in a short period of time. In Sri Lanka, the practice of this speciality is a challenge due to the gaps in infra-structure and a shortage of resources. As is the case in other resource-poor settings, infertility services are perceived to be of less priority when set against other more pressing problems such as infections and non-communicable diseases (Okonofua 1996). Additionally, the high fertility rate observed in Sri Lanka in the past may have undermined the development of infertility care. The total fertility rate (TFR), which dropped to 1.93 and hence fell below replacement fertility in the late 1990s (DCS and MOH 2000), has once again increased to 2.3 (DCS and MOH 2009) and has generated concerns over infertility care initiatives. The return of investment in terms of success in infertility treatments is disappointingly low when compared to other high-end, high-tech medical treatment modalities. Nonetheless, infertility has been noted to be a global health problem (WHO 2002) along with the unmet need for ARTs. As Ombelet argues in his chapter, assisted reproductive technologies should be made available to all who need them, irrespective of their social or economic status. Currently, in developing countries of the kind discussed here in Part II of the book, it is estimated that only 1 per cent of infertile couples receive appropriate ART treatment (Nachtigall 2006; Vayena et al. 2009). While Sri Lanka has had high-quality infertility treatment available for longer than many other countries of similar economic status, access still remains a major issue for all but the wealthiest.

In the past, infertile couples from Sri Lanka sought advanced infertility treatment at centres overseas such as those in India and Singapore. The high cost of such a strategy meant that this option was affordable to only a small minority. Many problems were also encountered by these couples on their return to Sri Lanka due to unforeseen complications and the clinical management of higher order multiple pregnancies. Such problems are not unique to Sri Lanka, and have been described elsewhere too (De Sutter 2011). The establishment of local ART services within the country in the late 1990s proved to be an important development as, for the first time, couples could get access to good quality services without the additional cost of overseas treatment and transport.

Globally, ARTs are a firmly regulated intervention in the provision of reproductive health care. Since the introduction of the

UK's Human Fertility and Embryology Act (HFEA) in 1990, the regulation of clinical and research work related to human embryos has been monitored and regulated by a recognised and competent authority. Many other countries have followed the UK model by introducing and implementing similar regulations and laws. In Sri Lanka, the National Science Foundation (NSF), under the Ministry of Science and Technology in collaboration with the Sri Lanka Medical Council (SLMC) initiated the introduction of regulations for the practice of ARTs in 2005. Experts from relevant fields were brought together and a 'provisional code of practice for assisted reproductive technologies' was developed for use by the centres providing this service (Sri Lanka Medical Council 2005). This exercise was taken further in 2009 as a draft bill to establish a regulatory body named the 'Human Reproduction and Genetics Authority' was formulated jointly by the NSF and the SLMC. Such an authority would be charged with overseeing all aspects of assisted reproductive technologies and work related to clinical genetics. The creation of such an authority is a significant breakthrough for Sri Lanka, since many other countries in the region as well as in the developing world lack such a system of regulations for ARTs. Clear regulations and a regulatory authority with legal powers are seen as integral to the development ARTs on a rational, scientific and ethical basis.

As with the practice of many other novel biotechnologies, public education about ARTs would do much to enhance their acceptance and development in the country. The high literacy rate in Sri Lanka has been considered an important factor when accounting for the high scores in regional health indicators that have been achieved over many years. Similarly, literacy rates are a factor in enabling clinicians to get across the complexities of 'informed choice' when undertaking ARTs as well as the types of infertility treatment that are now available. In spite of strong social and cultural beliefs, negative attitudes towards advanced treatment modalities have not been observed. Whereas infertility carries considerable stigma in Sri Lanka, treatments appear to be welcomed and given a strong public endorsement. High acceptance rates for ART have been observed among the medical profession (Dissanayake, Simpson and Jayasekara 2002; Simpson, Dissanayake and Jayasekara 2005). As Sri Lanka is a multicultural and multi-religious society the importance of identifying these differences has been emphasised in the way that regulatory frameworks have been developed (Seneviratne 2011). For example, concerns have been raised in clinical practice about the circumstances under which donor gametes might be used and how the sensitive issues this practice raises should be addressed in different communities (Inhorn 2009; an issue also discussed by several authors in this volume: Hudson and Culley; Tremayne; Clarke; Mahmoud).

In a resource-poor setting such as Sri Lanka, practitioners of assisted reproductive technologies face some unique challenges that are not faced by their counterparts in better-resourced health systems. Since centres in Sri Lanka are operated in the private sector, a competitive atmosphere prevails. While such competition may be conducive to the enhancement of services, it can sometimes have a negative impact. The faith invested in ARTs as a solution to infertility problems leads to client-driven non-medical indications for ART presenting at clinics. Ethically, what are in effect social and emotional issues should be explored initially through careful counselling, and only then should decisions be taken about technological intervention.

Informing the public of the facilities available is a duty of all practitioners. Likewise, corporate promotion is a necessity for any private sector enterprise. Establishing a balance between each of these pulls is a challenge in a resource-poor setting, and advertising needs to operate within the context of accepted norms for medical products and services. In the UK, the HFEA has adopted a policy of total disclosure of information about the services provided as this assures the rights of the clients and reduces the possibility of them being misled. However, the boundary between public information and advertising for self-promotion is unclear in Sri Lanka and regulations governing ART in Sri Lanka continue to find ways of addressing the issues. Unverified claims of the success and effectiveness of new investigations and treatment modalities are regularly reported in the media. These also present a challenge for local practitioners and need to be evaluated by the authority in the best interests of the public. While recognising that such media reports may broaden awareness among the public about advanced treatment options for infertility, it should also be noted that some have given rise to unrealistic expectations. In the absence of a regulatory authority with a remit for public understanding of ARTs, it remains in the hands of the practitioners in the field to use the media sensibly and ethically for the benefit of the public.

In resource-poor countries, the development of ARTs has been hampered by a lack of trained personnel. Currently this void in knowledge transfer is being filled by visiting experts from overseas as part of long-standing collaborations such as those that currently operate with Indian clinics. Recently, the PGIM has commenced sub-specialist training and board certification in subfertility. The curriculum includes areas such as pelvic surgery in advanced pelvic disease and the management of complications resulting from ART treatment. Although in the private sector ART centres provide up-to-date facilities, infrastructure development has yet to be adequately established in the government sector. Policy makers are, however, focusing their attention on this important area, as it is fast advancing.

As in other developing countries, the cost of ARTs is the single most important factor in relation to access to services. The mean monthly income of a household in Sri Lanka is estimated be around Rs.35,000 (£173 at the time of writing in June 2013) while the cost of an IVF treatment cycle is around Rs.400,000 (£1,980). This figure is close to the annual salary of an average couple. In comparison, the UK figures show the average monthly income to be around £2,100, while the cost of an IVF treatment cycle is around £3,500 – less than two months earnings for an average household. As the financial implications of undergoing ART in Sri Lanka are greater, so the expectations from a treatment cycle increase. Many Sri Lankans will use savings or personal belongings to raise the funds required for ART treatment. Awareness that ART would be the only opportunity for parenthood places added pressure on the couple as well as the practitioners. A reduction in cost would of course increase the number of people who could afford such treatment (Ombelet and Campo 2007) but treatment should be provided without compromises in the quality of care. Low-cost treatment plans should be adequately evaluated for their cost benefit prior to introduction into clinical practice. In a study conducted in Egypt, it was shown that over two-thirds of couples who underwent IVF treatment felt low-cost natural cycles are acceptable, in spite of the lower pregnancy rates (Shahin 2007). As low-cost ART treatments are still new in Sri Lanka, their efficacy is yet to be evaluated. A hope is that the advancement of such low-cost treatment modalities will one day make ARTs affordable to many lower-income couples in developed countries as well (*Nature* 2006).

Lack of other allied services in infertility care is a further shortcoming in Sri Lanka. The importance of services such as psychological counselling in care of the infertile couples is well recognised. Such services have been integrated into treatment preparation in some centres in the country, but many others have not included them. Whether the desired objectives of allied services are achieved in the presence of financial constraints is uncertain. It is often noted that couples decline post-treatment counselling following failure to achieve a viable conception, as they see no apparent benefit, only an added cost. There is a need therefore to integrate such services into the treatment package so patients would be able to understand and possibly benefit from their experience.

Greater research into infertility in the developing world would address problems specific to particular geographical areas and thereby improve diagnosis and treatment strategies, as disease patterns display wide variation. For example, tubal factor infertility, which is thought to be a major contributory factor in African countries affecting over 50 per cent of the infertile couples (Murage, Muteshi and Githae 2011), has been shown to affect less than 10 per cent in a study in Sri Lanka (Palihawadana, Wijesinghe and Seneviratne 2012). This figure could be explained by the low incidence of Sexually Transmitted Infections (STIs) such as Chlamydia Trachomatis infection, which has been shown to be present in less than 8 per cent in a Sri Lankan study (Palihawadana, Dissanayake, Harshani and Wijesinghe 2012). Consequently, the need for ARTs can be expected to be different in different countries. Further, the infrastructure facilities and staff available are dissimilar between regions and countries of the developing world. This heterogeneity should be recognised, indicating that a single model of providing services would not suit all countries that fall into the 'developing' category (Rutstein and Iqbal 2004).

In Sri Lanka, one priority is to develop low-cost ART techniques that would have the potential to benefit a much wider sector of the population, as recommended by an expert committee of the WHO (WHO 2002) and by Willem Ombelet (this volume). Natural cycle and minimal stimulation ART cycles along with newer stimulation regimes have been shown to reduce the cost of treatment (Noorashikin et al. 2008; Nargund 2009). This however has to be matched against the success rates of such treatment. An expansion of basic, clinical and applied research in ART in Sri Lanka is desirable. Research into clinical manifestation (Wijeyaratne et al. 2011), demography (Wijesinghe 2012) and clinical application of aetiology of polycystic ovarian syndrome (PCOS) (Seneviratne et al. 2009) have provided useful guidelines for ART use. As in all spheres of medicine, having the private sector as the main setting for providing ART limits the resources availability for academic and research activities. In future, the establishment of centres in academic settings such as universities would help to improve research as well as provide the leadership required to develop regulations and guidelines.

In terms of ethics, clinicians and policy makers face three fundamental dilemmas with regards to infertility care within Sri Lanka. First, the justification for the allocation of funds and other resources to ART services, when many other conditions such as communicable diseases and many non-communicable diseases still claim lives on a regular basis. Infertility, as a non-life threatening condition, tends to take lower priority in the allocation of a meagre health budget. Second, as in other successful areas of health care in Sri Lanka, the government has a responsibility to provide such services so that infertility services can benefit people from any socio-economic status, but it often lacks economic resources and political will. The third dilemma faced by clinicians centres on who should receive treatment and what treatment should be offered on the basis of factors affecting success and treatment complications. As in any part of the world where such services are provided, the clinicians are left to their own judgement when a woman of advanced age seeks ART or when a young couple seek such treatment prematurely for non-medical reasons, such as when a partner is about to leave for a long period of employment abroad. Since couples are likely to be financing their own treatment entirely, they might claim levels of reproductive autonomy which do not fully take into account future implications. In the UK, the HFEA currently advocates that such decisions are only made after consultation with clinicians and counsellors on an individual case basis, and taking the welfare of the possible child into consideration. Such concepts are also adopted in Sri Lanka, though a satisfactory monitoring system has yet to be established.

Conclusion and Cross-Cutting Themes

In providing this brief overview of fertility treatments in Sri Lanka we would like to draw attention to five key themes that emerge here, and that reflect themes raised in the other chapters in this part.

High Levels of Endorsement of ARTs

Reproductive disruption experienced in the context of economically developing countries brings with it considerable social pressure and a deep-seated sense of stigma. The motivation for couples to seek out treatment is therefore high and is often driven by a sense of desperation, which brings emotional, social and health problems in its wake. Against this backdrop, ARTs are often welcomed and there is considerable investment in the idea that advanced technologies can solve all infertility problems.

Access

Structural factors in the health sector have a significant impact on access to treatment. Governments endeavour to provide basic infertility services, however, the pace of technological advance and the costs of new therapies means that services are unevenly distributed and many have no hope of access. As in Sri Lanka, ARTs mostly appear in the private sector and only years later, if at all, in the public sector. Typically, the public sector lags a long way behind the leading edge of infertility treatment in the private sector. Indeed, as the Sri Lankan example shows, some private sector provision in economically developing countries can be on a par with services anywhere in the world. However, investment in infertility treatments is often seen as a low priority when pitched against broader health objectives such as disease control, vaccination and other public health initiatives. As the chapter by Willem Ombelet demonstrates, low-income thresholds and the politics of access to ARTs are closely entwined. He points out that ARTs remain available to a very small proportion of the world's population, despite the burden of involuntary childlessness being particularly heavy in low-income settings. Seeking to shift the tenor of discussion, Ombelet argues that infertility should be considered as a public health issue, rather than simply an individual medical problem as it is in parts of the Global North.

Knowledge Transfer

An important aspect of the availability of ARTs in developing world settings is the transfer of knowledge and expertise to carry out highly specialist treatments. Access to ARTs in economically developing countries typically begins either with foreign teams delivering treatments locally or with people travelling abroad to other parts of Asia, Europe or the United States for treatment. Either way, this means that treatments are only available to the very richest in society. However, over time, local expertise develops and services can be accessed without the need to bring in costly teams from overseas or engage in expensive overseas travel. As this chapter demonstrates, knowledge begins to be embedded among a wider network of local practitioners who are then able to press for better resources and improve access to specialised treatment.

Regulation

Despite being an area of biomedicine that excites considerable interest and controversy, the growth of ARTs in economically developing countries typically occurs before any regulatory frameworks are in place to deal with what practitioners are actually doing. Consequently, we argue, there is a good deal of self-regulation in place in the ART sector. Governments often find themselves playing 'catch-up' and, usually in the face of scandal or abuse, have to resort to regulatory fixes that draw on frameworks taken from countries that appear to be further down the road to effective regulation. This is the case in Sri Lanka, where HFEA guidelines have been particularly influential.

Complexity of Integration

In all the examples presented in Part II, ARTs do not make their appearance into a vacuum. On the contrary, doctors and patients practise in settings that are marked by long-standing beliefs, assumptions and practices about reproduction, gender, health and well-being, misfortune and fate. As the studies of Bangladesh [Nahar], Mali [Hörbst] and Botswana [Bochow] presented here show, the assimilation of ARTs is a complex process that has to be understood in terms of the prevailing social and cultural norms in each country setting.

Thilina S. Palihawadana MB BS(Col), MRCOG(UK), MPhil(Col), MSc in Clin Embryology (Leeds) is a senior lecturer in reproductive biology at the Faculty of Medicine, University of Kelaniya, Sri Lanka. He has published widely on infertility and ARTs in developing world countries.

H.R. Seneviratne MBBS(Ceylon), DM (Col), FCOG (Sri Lanka), FRCOG (UK) is a retired senior professor of obstetrics and gynaecology, University of Colombo, Sri Lanka. He is the founder of the Vindana Reproductive Health Centre, Colombo, and a pioneer of IVF treatment Sri Lanka.

PART III

ARTs and Professional Practice

Part III – Introduction

ETHNIC COMMUNITIES, PROFESSIONS AND PRACTICES

Alison Shaw

As a contribution to the discussion of the moral worlds of 'ethnic communities, professionals and practitioners' in the context of new reproductive technologies, here I offer some comments that are intended to highlight the significance of the two chapters in this part, and to point to some of the connections between them.

The phrase 'ethnic communities' itself tends to conjure up or reinforce the idea that there are compartmentalised moral worlds, located in spheres neatly demarcated according to ancestry, religion, culture and social positioning. It pertains particularly to 'minorities' in societies where the concept of ethnicity is both a tool for monitoring racism, exclusion and disadvantage, and a means of political and socio-economic leverage. Statistically, it can be said that ethnic minorities exist. Yet the concept of ethnicity is fragile and liable to dissolve. Ethnicity can evoke a community constructed through sharing a heritage, language, religion and way of life, and promoted both through state discourse and the activities of its representatives, but it can also disintegrate when its components are scrutinised. I wonder how informative 'ethnicity' is likely to continue to be now that more than half of British 'South Asians' and 'black Caribbeans' are born in Britain, inter-ethnic partnerships are common, and having mixed parentage is increasingly likely.

In the context of health and welfare provision, ethnicity data provide one of various means of tracking inequalities in service use and health outcomes. 'Cultural competence' training is one strategy aimed at improving minority access to health care and thus reducing these inequalities, by instilling in health professionals 'cross-cultural skills' and 'cultural sensitivity'. It is based on the assumption that 'culture' refers to diversity in personal values and ways of life that are sufficiently systematic to indicate group and not just individual characteristics. The problem is that when incorporated into policy and practice, this view of culture often translates into a compendium of group characteristics of an ethnic minority that are assumed to differ uniformly from the majority and apply uniformly to the minority. Stereotyping of this sort overlooks within-group diversity and the allegiances, interests and effects of social and cultural change that cut across ethnic identities.

To exercise 'cultural competence' without emphasising boundaries and difference requires health professionals to develop generic skills that will empower them to work with a diversity of patients, for such is the reality of health care in complex societies. Factual information about the main socio-economic, cultural, religious and linguistic dimensions of diversity is important, but it is not sufficient because professionals also need to be empowered to respond to patients as individuals. This entails a sort of moral imagination: 'this person belongs to a particular ethnic group – as she has told me, or as it says on her records, or as I know from her name – and I know that this might mean she holds values different from mine and so she might respond to a particular treatment option in a way that I might not – but I cannot assume this, I need to find out'. And moral imagination is, in turn, linked to socio-cultural self-awareness – an awareness that one's own values and practices are socially constructed, and that on the basis of these constructions we tend to project assumptions about how the values of practices of other people differ, especially if those people are visibly different from ourselves.

In the first chapter in this part, 'Reproductive Technologies and Ethnic Minorities: Beyond a Marginalising Discourse on the Marginalised Communities', Sangeeta Chattoo addresses this aspect of cultural competency. She examines the views of oncology health professionals about their patients' responses to being informed that cancer treatment may threaten their fertility and learning that there are fertility 'preservation' options available.

Chattoo shows that health professionals tend to assume that 'culture' and 'religion' rather than personal choices shape South Asian patients' responses to information about infertility and its management, whereas white patients are assumed to respond as autonomous individuals, in 'culture-free' ways. Two generalisations about South Asians are common: one is that the patriarchal family denies autonomy to adult children; the other is that South Asian families are strongly pro-natalist and consequently 'secretive' about fertility problems, because knowledge of compromised fertility is likely to undermine the practice of arranging marriages. In the light of these assumptions about South Asian culture, health professionals may think that even discussing fertility treatment with such patients is strongly 'taboo' or at least liable to cause offence, and so they may be inclined to withhold information from patients. This amounts to a discriminatory stance that if translated into practice undermines the principle of informed choice regarding medical treatment.

Chattoo's examples show that these kinds of professional generalisations about South Asians are frequently based on half-truths and imperfect knowledge, or on exceptional cases, or straightforward prejudice. It is common, for example, for women – or women plus their partners – from all ethnic groups initially to refuse oncology treatment if it will compromise fertility; in general, information about compromised fertility is painful to accept and difficult to negotiate, and more nuanced responses may take time. Another example concerns prevailing stereotypes about South Asian extended families, which reflect imperfect knowledge of diversity in family forms and household structure, and are additionally founded upon false inferences about what South Asian kinship entails in the context of health care.

The stereotypical 'traditional' South Asian family is something like this: a corporate several-generational entity comprising a senior couple with their married sons and the sons' wives and children living under one roof; it is hierarchically organised by gender and age, and decisions are ultimately approved or vetoed by the household head or senior couple. In Britain, some South Asian households correspond approximately to this picture at some points of their lifecycle, but the results of surveys investigating change in marriage patterns and household formation in Britain show that today's typical British nuclear family, comprising a couple and their children, is more likely to be of South Asian than of white or black Caribbean ethnicity (Berthoud 2005). Moreover, although South

Asians have lower rates of divorce and separation, and show a less marked turn from the 'traditional' British nuclear family towards lone-parenthood and family reconstitution, there are indications of a shift in perceptions of arranged marriages – which have long-been contrasted with 'love' marriages in another 'us–them' stereotype – and changes in the expectations of conjugality and marriage (Qureshi, Charsley and Shaw 2012).

When accessing fertility treatment, the idea that South Asians live with extended family gives rise to another stereotype: that other members of a South Asian extended household will have a stake in a woman or couple's fertility – being, according to stereotype, pro-natalists who arrange their children's marriages – and so will necessarily be involved in decisions about medical treatment that potentially compromises fertility, as well as in decisions about infertility treatment. This image of the South Asian family as, in Chattoo's phrase, 'a seamless moral unit', implies two further, somewhat contradictory assumptions. Chattoo delineates one of these as 'a culture of silence and deceit', whereby a desire to avoid sharing details about use of assisted reproductive technologies with extended family members (that would, for other patients, be understood as a desire for confidentiality) is reinterpreted for South Asians pathologically – 'confidentiality' rephrased as 'secrecy' is too easily interpreted as 'deceit', even though desire for donor secrecy continues to be important for couples, regardless of their ethnicity. The relationship with household structure is more a practical matter, since maintaining confidentiality about personal information can pose practical challenges that clinicians might need to be aware of – for instance, concerning letters and telephone calls relaying clinical information. The other assumption about the extended family as a corporate entity, even when its members may be living in separate households, is that health information will be more easily shared within it; but this too is problematic, as research on the disclosure of genetic risk information has shown. Such information may or may not be shared for a range of reasons, which includes the desire not to cause needless emotional distress (Shaw 2009; Shaw and Hurst 2009).

The chapter also shows how awareness of cultural difference can be a source of anxiety for health professionals. There is concern that they might, unwittingly, suggest someone breaks a religious prohibition when they open discussions with South Asians about such techniques as gamete retrieval, donor insemination or sperm banking. In fact, such fears may be completely irrelevant: a man might decline sperm banking or a couple might resist donor insemination not on religious grounds, but for personal reasons. Clinicians are professionally obliged to raise these options; to fail to do so, on grounds of assumed religious or cultural sensitivities, would be discriminatory, potentially resulting in treatment options not being openly discussed, and then treatment being requested or declined without fully informed consideration. Chattoo's final example illustrates the complexity of these issues. It is an extract from an interview with an oncology nurse specialist who reflects on the case of a young Pakistani Muslim woman who declined a hysterectomy after her cancer had spread. This nurse specialist does not make essentialist assumptions about culture and religion. While the nursing team assumed that the young woman's treatment decision was made for religious reasons and the pressures of an arranged marriage, the nurse specialist felt that the young woman's decision was indeed her own – but she remains unsure whether she is right or wrong in not treating South Asians any differently from anyone else. The nurse specialist's point indicates the need to build professional confidence in working with cultural diversity without resorting to essentialism.

The second chapter in this part, by Nicky Hudson and Lorraine Culley, considers the implications of the views of British South Asians on the moral dilemmas raised by third-party egg and sperm donation for understanding diversity in attitudes to and use of fertility treatment. Their chapter, 'Knock, Knock, "You're my Mummy": Anonymity, Identification and Gamete Donation in British South Asian Communities', is focused on the issues raised by donor anonymity. In the UK since 2005, gamete donation has ceased to be anonymous in that a child conceived as a consequence of donation has a legal right, after the age of 18, to receive information about their donor parent. The impact of this on donor recruitment is a matter of debate, but there remains a shortage of donors in the UK in general, and especially from ethnic-minority backgrounds. The result is inequitable opportunities for fertility treatment using donor gametes.

Hudson and Culley's chapter investigates the willingness of British South Asians to donate eggs and sperm. In particular, it interrogates the suggestion that South Asian men and women are less willing, for cultural and religious reasons, to donate gametes than whites, and more willing to use known or family donors. Their study participants comprised in total one hundred British South Asian men and women of Indian, Pakistani and Bangladeshi origins. These participants had never themselves received fertility treatment or acted as donors, and were of diverse ages. They were invited to engage in ethical reflection upon the acceptability and potential impact of 'identifiable' gamete donation within their respective ethnic communities.

Initially, the study participants' attitudes to gamete donation were, in general, favourable. They recognised that gamete donation would be a strategy of last resort and be likely to invoke social disapproval, and many of the Muslims felt it would raise religious concerns, but despite this, the South Asian study participants viewed fertility treatment by gamete donation as an altruistic means of easing the suffering of childless couples. However, on being informed about the removal of donor anonymity, the study participants raised specific concerns. These concerns were quite clearly gendered, but cut across ethnicity and religion. Men and women across the study sample additionally felt that the potential repercussions of non-anonymity through the wider family and community rendered 'identifiable' donation too risky.

Hudson and Culley observe that numerous other studies have noted gender differences in views about gamete donation, but none has elaborated on the particular ways in which, in this study, women were seen as emotionally connected to donor-conceived children by means of their donated biogenetic material. Specifically, women worried about the potential emotional turmoil that non-anonymity could bring them and their families in the future. There was also concern that non-anonymity could result in male donors becoming financially responsible for future offspring identified as theirs. The authors note that this concern derives from the strong link, for Muslims, between biological paternity and the inheritance of property, as Islamic rules of inheritance are based on patrilineal blood ties. It is to protect the connection between perceived biological lineage and the inheritance of property that Islam prohibits formal legal adoption in the Western sense whereby a non-biological child can acquire all the rights and duties of a biological child (Atighetchi 2007: 139–40). The Sikhs and Hindus in the sample also felt that sperm donation was more problematic than egg donation, but saw this as cultural rather than religious; for them, it was a consequence of the social importance of fatherhood, male lineage and genetic paternity for a person's social and biological identity in South Asian societies. This observation resonates with a substantial ethnographic literature documenting the importance in South Asia of patrilineal descent for how people construct their identities, their notions of belonging, their projections of the past and the future, and their understandings of biological inheritance (Böck and Rao 2000). Indeed, such notions are relevant across South Asia and parts of Europe through to the Middle East and North Africa (King and Stone 2010). This is good example of how culture and religion may signify in self-representations, as well as in representations constructed by academics and by health professionals.

Hudson and Culley then suggest that the 'shared tradition of intra-family adoption', a practice that their study participants reported as being a South Asian cultural tradition, might offer a solution to the shortage of South Asian gamete donors. Informal adoption within families is sometimes practised as a solution to childlessness in South Asia, and most of the participants in Hudson and Culley's study had heard of this practice. Usually it involves a 'family decision': a couple who already have children may decide, or be requested by a senior relative, to give their next baby to a childless couple – thus, a son and his wife could give a baby to a childless brother and his wife, the child remaining within the extended family network. Extrapolating from this, the participants in Hudson and Culley's study considered egg or sperm donation within the family as a theoretically parallel practice, involving the 'same' biogenetic material. But they were also aware of the potentially problematic aspects of both practices. This concerned the social and emotional risk to the parents of a child 'donated' by informal adoption or conceived through family-donated gametes of losing the child in the future. This could happen if the child were to choose one day to return to his or her donor/genetic parent(s), or if the donor parent(s) were subsequently to claim the child. Additionally, they felt that inter-family gamete donation could easily be seen as a transgression of the norm that reproduction occurs within marriage.

The ethical reflections of Hudson and Culley's research participants thus caution against assuming that intra-family gamete donation would be a 'culturally appropriate' treatment strategy for infertile South Asian couples, given the shortage of South Asian donors. There is a cultural essentialism embedded in the idea that specific services are appropriate or necessary for particular ethnic or religious communities; the reality is that attitudes to reproductive options vary within and between ethnic groups, and change over time (Sheikh and Esmail 2007; Shaw 2011). And it is in the light of this variation, as well as in the light of ethical and clinical factors, that specific options within a range of services will be appropriate or necessary for some users of health care and not others. For instance, besides the ethical considerations, the fact that siblings share biogenetic material would require clinicians to rule out any genetic factors underlying unsuccessful reproduction in the case of fertile but childless couples for whom intra-family gamete donation might be a 'last resort' strategy. More generally, the discussion of 'identifiable' gamete donation points to the need for further cross-ethnic national and international research into the long-term social and ethical implications of third-party gamete donation.

Considered together, these two chapters offer a reminder that 'ethnic communities' do not consist of people inhabiting culturally bounded moral worlds. In the context of health care access and delivery for a multi-ethnic society, the idea of cultural diversity offers an approximate tool for monitoring and addressing inequalities. Cultural competence is not about denying difference but about ensuring equality of access to health care options. Cultural awareness is about being sensitive to the social and cultural shaping of the moral worlds we all inhabit, and recognising that on some dimensions ethnic differences both exist and are cross-cut by within-group variation and social and generational change (see Simpson, Blell and Hampshire, this volume). A particular individual response might be more likely than another but can never be assumed, and the main dimensions of ethnic diversity cannot be reduced to cultural inventories or 'us–them' dichotomies. In short, cultural competence requires treating patients as individuals, on a case-by-case basis, ensuring that, in each case, clinically relevant treatment options are offered and considered, and accepted or rejected.

The chapters in Part III thus offer valuable insights for raising awareness of the ways in which ideas about 'ethnic communities' as socio-cultural and ethno-religious entities are both reinforced and challenged in the day-to-day experiences and imaginings of medical and social science professionals, patients, and members of the general public as they engage in ethical reflection on the use of techniques of assisted reproduction.

Alison Shaw is a senior research fellow in social anthropology at the University of Oxford. Her research interests are in ethnicity, ethnic diversity and health; medical anthropology/sociology;

social aspects of genetics/genomics; kinship, gender and transnational marriages; South Asian Islam/Islam in Europe and Islamic bioethics. She has done fieldwork in Pakistan and in the UK. She has completed several research projects with British Pakistani families, updating her first fieldwork by tracing marriage patterns in the second and third generations.

Chapter 10

REPRODUCTIVE TECHNOLOGIES AND ETHNIC MINORITIES

BEYOND A MARGINALISING DISCOURSE ON THE MARGINALISED COMMUNITIES

Sangeeta Chattoo

This chapter will offer a critique of the emerging field of the use of assisted reproductive technologies (ARTs) by minority ethnic communities in the UK. I will argue that, given the semantic underpinnings of 'ethnicity' as a euphemism for race/racisms, exclusion and discrimination within the context of health and social care, and its conflation with 'minority' 'communities', the field created by the inter-space of the three terms pre-empts a marginalising discourse on the marginalised, reinforcing essentialised perceptions of cultural and religious difference. The numerical notion of a 'minority' seeks to naturalise rather than challenge the underlying structural issues of partial citizenship (see Brah 1996; Hesse and Sayyid 2006; Chattoo and Atkin 2012). Paradoxically, the need to focus on exclusion and disadvantage has only relocated these groups to the political and social margins of the state; reproducing individual subjects as passive victims of their social positioning (for a conceptual debate on the state and its margins, see Das and Poole 2004: 3–34). I argue that 'ethnicity' does not create an analytical space within which we can analyse how individuals negotiate or resist such constructions or loci of power represented by community, state, health and social care organisations in negotiating infertilities and the use of New Reproductive Technologies (NRTs).

This is not to deny the contribution of critical theorists who have used political debates on ethnicity and race to remind us of the fragile boundaries of an ideal liberal, democratic state (Modood 1997, 2008; Kumar 2008). Nor is it to ignore the work of post-colonial feminist writers on intersectionality between, race, gender, ethnicity and class (Anthias and Yuval-Davis 1992; Phoenix 2009; Mirza 2010), and the sophisticated writings of post-modernist theorists on negotiation of multiple and diasporic identities within different socio-political contexts (see Bhabha 1994; Baumann 1997; Werbner 1997). None of these debates however seem to inform policy and practice discourses on ethnicity and health in the UK, which continue to treat people of minority ethnic backgrounds as homogenised conglomerates of culture, religion and tradition (Lo and Stacey 2008). At the same time, there is nonetheless a policy imperative towards providing culturally competent care across countries in the West (Bhui et al. 2007). While the implicit aim of such policies is to redress inequities in access to health and social care, there are obvious tensions here with a wider policy focus on individual choice and patient-centred care, to which I return. The common response to recognising difference takes the form of standardised protocols, often developed in consultation with (self-selected) community and religious leaders. Such bureaucratic responses to ethnic and religious diversity often attempt to provide simplified solutions to a fundamentally complex challenge faced by any modern, liberal democracy (see Taylor 1994).

The crux of the challenge lies in the fact that health and welfare provision in any multi-ethnic society, by definition, involves contested plural social and religious values regarding the relationship between individual, family and state, as well as wider legal definitions of the democratic rights and duties of citizens in relation to those of the state (Law 2003). Hence, there is bound to be debate on, and resistance towards, default social and legal values, often representing a dominant majority, by people of non-majority ethnic groups (Bauman 1992), in addition to internal contestations on social values within any ethnic community (Das 1995; Baumann 1997). This chapter argues that in order to understand and address the goal of culturally competent care within the field of ARTs, we need to destabilise the notions of ethnicity, community and culture by focusing on how health care professionals constitute these terms within their every day practice.

The following two sections of the chapter will focus on unpicking the notion of ethnicity within health care research and practice, and the assumptions underpinning the notion of 'culturally competent care'. These sections will be followed by some examples from empirical research to highlight the engagements of health professionals with people from minority ethnic backgrounds.

Why Destabilise the Notion of Ethnicity?

In destabilising the notion of ethnicity, a case will be made for shifting the discourse on ethnicity and reproductive technologies from the margins of a specialised academic and policy discourse to the centre of a theory of modern social life and identity, as suggested by Fenton (2003). From a social science perspective, ethnicity is best defined as a field of inquiry that helps us to identify the material and cultural context within which ethnic identities, premised on notions of nationality, heritage, religion and language, are constantly redefined and contested by different social groups. Importantly, there is often an intersection between the concepts of 'ethnic group', race and nation that shares an emphasis on a notion of common descent and culture (for excellent case studies, see the volume edited by Wade 2007). That is to say, ethnicity does not refer to a theoretical concept with a predefined content. Rather, in Fenton's terms, 'ethnicity refers to the social construction of descent and culture, the social mobilisation of descent and culture, and the meanings and implications of the classification systems built around them. People or peoples do not just possess cultures or share ancestry; *they elaborate these into the idea of a community founded upon these attributes*' (Fenton 2003: 3, original emphasis).

Following on from the above, culture and community do not refer to innate or inherited attributes that people 'have', but rather to dynamic processes of self-identity and differentiation involving negotiation of boundaries of inclusion, exclusion and struggles over power and resources between groups (Hall 1996). Consequently, dominant voices within ethnic groups as a collective often project a cohesive image of their culture, community, religion and kinship forms (Anderson 1991). As cautioned by Baumann (1997), we need to differentiate between dominant and demotic (alternate) voices within a community, keeping the descriptive and analytical concepts apart. Hence, while we know that ethnicity is an abstraction that connotes descent, country of origin, religion, culture, and linguistic and nationalistic affiliations among other things, researchers often fail to identify the specific context used within analysis (Bradby 2003). Operationalising ethnicity and culture (the specific meaning we attribute to the term within a context), is the first step before we can help to address the complexity and dilemmas of providing culturally competent care. Before I turn to the empirical part of the chapter, it is important to look at the notion of cultural competence a bit more critically.

Why Engage more Critically with the Notion of Cultural Competence?

At a broader level, it is important to recognise a complex conflation between ethnicity and socio-economic position in relation to indices of health and health outcomes for a majority of minoritised ethnic groups (see Nazroo 2001, 2003; Karlsen, Becares and Roth 2012). There is considerable evidence suggesting that health and social care professionals often fail to provide accessible and appropriate care to people from minority ethnic backgrounds, either ignoring or misrepresenting their needs (Chattoo et al. 2002; Bhui et al. 2007; Rouse 2009; Culley and Hudson 2009b; Atkin and Anionwu 2010). Equitable and culturally appropriate health and social care provision remains a major challenge within the context of a rapidly changing demographic profile and shifting boundaries of minority and majority communities in certain parts of England (such as Leicester and London), as reflected in the 2001 census. An increasing number of children are born and brought up within families of mixed ethnic origins with plural cultural/religious identities. This has particular significance for how we rethink the relationship between ethnicity and nationality for diasporic communities. Further, it poses the question: how can social science perspectives help us to achieve the goal of 'culturally competent care' within an ethnically diverse society, in which 50 per cent of people of immigrant origin have, in fact, been born in the UK?

As social scientists, we should be concerned with what constitutes 'evidence' and who is producing it for pedagogical practices related to cultural competency. At the surface, according to trainers of health, nursing and social work professionals, the basic components of models of cultural competency cover three areas: cultural sensitivity, cultural knowledge and cultural skills (Kim-Godwin, Clarke and Barton 2001). However, each component assumes a static notion of culture as a shared system of beliefs and values or worldview that can be described and 'known' in order to be incorporated into short training courses for health and social care professionals. A focus on 'diversity management' within health care settings often translates into another bureaucratic exercise, codifying religious and cultural difference without helping professionals to deal with the complexity and heterogeneity of beliefs and experiences within, or similarities across, ethnic and religious groups.

Gunaratnam (2008: 25), using Giddens' notion of an 'abstract system',[1] suggests that such attempts at regulating practice and responses to caring can lead to 'sequestration of experience', and 'undermine equity and erode responsibility for emotional and moral thinking through their attempts to simplify and control the threat of the unfamiliar'. However, she also shows how individual health care professionals challenge such attempts at codification of responses in their negotiations of the emotional complexities of the lives of the individuals they are caring for, reinscribing uncertainties and dilemmas posed by caring within the context of old age and death. This serves as a reminder that professionals as individuals also have different subject positions, and even though their response and practices of care are governed by a code of professional culture/ethics, in practice, the values underpinning these are interpreted and negotiated differently by individuals (see Chattoo and Atkin 2009). Let me provide a few examples from my research to highlight how health and social care professionals engage with people from South Asian backgrounds. I want to focus on how standardised notions of cultural competence are threatened by a lurking presence of generalisations and personal views about particular communities as homogenous aggregates, and how the visibility of difference redraws the boundaries between self and the 'immigrant-settler' as 'unknown'. I will first provide a brief note on the research context and method.

A Note on Research Context and Method

I am using material from a larger, two-year qualitative project (for details, see Chattoo, Crawshaw and Atkin 2010) that explored the social implications of threats to fertility caused by treatment for cancer, faced by adults diagnosed with cancer. The project involved in-depth interviews with forty-seven participants (twenty-nine men and eighteen women) between 18 and 40 years of age, from South Asian (Indian, Pakistani and Bangladeshi) and white (majority and minority) backgrounds, who had undergone invasive treatment for cancer. Some had been diagnosed in childhood or early teens. It is important to bear in mind the specific therapeutic context of cancer within which threats to fertility were experienced and negotiated by men and women differently. Following guidelines provided by the National Institute for Clinical Excellence (NICE 2005) and the Royal College of Physicians, the Royal College of Radiologists, and the Royal College of Obstetricians and Gynaecologists (RCP, RCR, RCOG 2007), the potential impact of treatment on fertility and appropriate 'preservation' (i.e. storing sperm, eggs or embryos) options should be discussed with teenagers and young adults. Clinical discussions and negotiations of *potential* threats and 'preservation' are marked by a dialectic of uncertainty and hope, since the impact on fertility is only revealed later. Young adults and teenagers thus confront profound questions of life, procreation and death, and potential 'forced choices' or 'non-choices' as suggested by Franklin (1997: 108) within the context of both storing (called 'banking') of gametes as well as potential use of assisted reproductive technologies (ARTs) in the future. In practice, given the pragmatics of technology (retrieval of sperm as opposed to eggs or embryos), a majority of women were not offered a choice.

The research also included three focus group discussions with seventeen professionals, and in-depth interviews with sixteen professionals representing oncology, reproductive medicine and social work. Out of the thirty-three professionals, twelve were from different minority ethnic backgrounds (including Indian, Pakistani, Iraqi, Polish, Hungarian, Irish and Scottish). This chapter is largely based on analysis of how professionals engaged with ideas of culture, religion and ethnicity within their everyday practice. However, where appropriate, references will be made to the experiences of participants who had undergone treatment.

The research was carried out with the help of three NHS trusts at three sites across England (North, Central and South) with a significant proportion of people from minority ethnic backgrounds, though the ethnic mix of populations was different at each site. The interviews and focus group discussions were carried out by three members of the research team and, at times, demonstrated slightly different styles of guiding the conversations.[2]

Why Focus on Professional Perspectives on Minoritised Communities?

It is not my intention to project a view of professionals as a homogenous whole. At the outset, the different disciplinary backgrounds of professionals working within oncology and reproductive medicine reflected different priorities. Specialists within oncology focused on starting treatment as soon as possible in order to achieve the best results and save lives, while specialists in reproductive medicine prioritised fertility preservation. Here, I am first interested in highlighting how professional reflections on issues of reproduction and the potential use of NRTs are interwoven with judgements about culture in terms of family life (gender and intergenerational values) and conjugality marking difference. These reflections cross-cut the boundaries between the public and the private domains of a patient's life (see Plumner 2003). Second, I want to analyse how notions of culture and religion are formulated in relation to people of South Asian backgrounds, in contrast with the emphasis on individuals and choice in discussions about patients from a white background (white minorities are not visible in these discussions). Such essentialised views on culture, community and gender are equally reinforced by professionals from minority ethnic backgrounds, an issue reserved for another discussion (Atkin and Chattoo 2007).

Professional Perceptions of South Asian Patients: The Tyranny of Family and Culture

One of the first stories that I heard at a fieldwork site meeting was about how 'Asian parents' intervene and prevent any discussion on issues related to fertility in consultations preceding treatment. While an open discussion on issues of sexuality and fertility between children and parents (especially of opposite sexes) might be a matter of embarrassment and intergenerational deference in particular families, the reference here was more specifically to the tradition of arranged marriages within 'Asian' communities, as pointed out later by one of the specialist nurses in her interview:

'... usually at the arranged marriage stage, because they don't want the new family to be aware that there might be an infertility problem. So we've certainly had that before, that this is a taboo subject; we are not to talk about it because it might scupper their chances of a good match' (FPR9).

The generalisation referred more specifically to young women from a Pakistani (Mirpuri region) Muslim community, without qualifying specific personal or family circumstances or how the young women might actively negotiate these arrangements within families. For example, FPR9 found it unusual that a 17- to 18-year-old girl was keen on having an ovarian function test before her parents started looking for a match:

> Well ..., her older sister ..., they were in the process of planning her marriage. She felt that she would be next. She didn't want to go into her arranged marriage without knowing definitely 'yes' or 'no' whether she was fertile, and she wanted her assessment so that she could be upfront with her future husband and say, you know, 'Yes, I want to get married but you have to know this beforehand'. She wasn't keen for her parents to know that she was going to have that done. So that was one, one case which I found very interesting.

At the meeting (mentioned above), there was also a suggestion that some young women are prevented by 'patriarchal families' from having treatment for cancer, since it is seen as jeopardising their chances of an arranged marriage. When pressed for details, it seemed that these storylines were based on half-true anecdotes that circulated like rumours in a team, leading to generalisations about culture and community. I will come back to the specific details about one such case. One of the oncologists later conceded that, within some families of Pakistani origin, the discussion on treatment of younger, unmarried women can be a bit protracted. This, of course, is very different from the initial suggestion (from another oncologist) that some patriarchal 'Asian' parents actively intervene to prevent their daughters from having treatment, so as not to jeopardise their chances of an arranged marriage. The possibility that a young woman might wish to trade off her survival for preserving her fertility, by choice, was overshadowed by the construction of her location within a stereotyped patriarchal family. Indeed, as suggested by a senior oncologist, it is not uncommon for young women from across ethnic backgrounds to disregard survival and treatment advice at diagnosis (Thewes et al. 2003: 508; Adams 2007). However, they are likely to give in under pressure of professional persuasion or a crisis brought on by the spread/recurrence of cancer. Such conflicting perceptions about treatment or gamete preservation are often constituted as examples or limitations of individual choice rather than as reflecting strong values of pro-natalism within white culture/s.

Out of the eighteen women, I came across only one (who happened to be of African-Portuguese origin) who had initially refused treatment since she was keen on having a family. This speaks of an association of womanhood with motherhood that cuts across ethnic groups, a similarity acknowledged by most professional participants in the study (Letherby 1999; Inhorn and Van Balen 2002; Throsby 2004). As summarised by one of the oncology specialist nurses (FG1) in a group discussion, 'I think, there's just similar feeling of loss. I get the same sort of sense of loss and devastation ... and deep feelings ... certainly from the women'. However, across and within cultures, there are alternate modes of dealing with and reconciling to such loss (Riessman 2002; Sandelowski and de Lacey 2002), given a biographical context. None of the five women of South Asian origin, two of whom were already married at the time of diagnosis, shared experiences of a repressive family or pressures to 'keep producing sons'. Only one of them (of Punjabi-Indian origin), in her early thirties, knew for certain that she could not have children. She and her (white) partner had never been keen on having a family and chose to remain 'childfree', after having briefly contemplated egg donation on the gynaecologist's suggestion. This is not to deny the presence of 'greater visibility' of infertility in South Asian communities (Culley and Hudson 2009b), where issues of conjugality and reproduction assume a collective ownership, especially within the context of an extended family structure (see Bharadwaj 2003; Hampshire, Blell and Simpson 2012a).

It might be a truism to state that rather than determining a norm, religion and gender within any culture set the boundaries of what is acceptable and not acceptable. Further, how individuals across ethnic groups negotiate such emotionally painful and ethically challenging decisions relate to a particular biography and an engagement with the notion of risk (both in terms of confronting cancer and their own mortality at a young age, and as a threat to fertility). Such engagements with risk and potential use of reproductive technologies lean on competing cultural discourses, including the one introduced by medicine. This is not to deny that, structurally, family, marriage and kinship or the relationship between self and community, or self and state, might operate differently across different ethnic or religious groups (cf. Das 1995).

As suggested earlier, both the therapeutic context of a life-threatening illness and the younger age profile of the participants in this research provide a varied landscape of life circumstances, reflecting complex negotiations of issues of reproduction and threats to fertility. Importantly, the sample included a small number of men and women who had made a choice not to pursue fertility treatment. A majority of the participants of South Asian origin were born and/or brought up in England, except two who had moved in the previous five to eight years following marriage, and one young man who was seeking asylum. Only two (Pakistani origin) couples lived as part of an extended family including parent/s and (unmarried) siblings (one did not have any children of their own and the other was recently married); while two other couples with children (of Pakistani, and Mauritian-Indian origins) lived with the husband's and wife's parents respectively. This picture is different from the static professional view of 'Asians' living in large extended family structures, dominated by patriarchal parents, where conjugality is defined by reproduction (through the male line), and excluding any notion of choice or romantic love – a theme to which I shall return.

It is interesting how quite contrary responses to treatment-related threats to fertility within families of South Asian background were equally attributed to strong pro-natalist values within their culture, without specifying religion, socio-economic background, individual or family circumstances. Thus, discussions about fertility were either perceived as a taboo for the over-protective 'Asian' parents or they were seen as pushing ethical boundaries (of autonomy) to preserve the fertility of their children. One of the specialists in reproductive medicine, for instance, was talking about a consultation regarding sperm banking with a young boy (over sixteen) who was seriously ill at the time. He found it awkward to have the discussion in the presence of his parents who, with their son's consent, insisted on sitting in and seemed (inappropriately in his opinion) to put equal weight on his fertility and recovery from cancer:

> [T]he patient was quite ill so wasn't making much of a response, and the parents were asking all the questions. It's very difficult to focus on the patient. And the impression they gave, they were as concerned about him sperm banking as they were about him – I mean

> the, the cancer – because of you know, grandchildren and things like that ... You do get the feeling that, culturally, the South Asian men, there is pressure to produce children. (MPR2)

Like other professionals, he conceded that parents often want to sit in on consultations of young people. This 'extreme case' just happened to involve a South Asian boy and, hence, stayed in his memory. What is striking about this excerpt is that, despite the young man's poor health, the clinical protocol introduced a 'choice' that he was not able to engage with. There was no discussion on the wider pro-natalist cultural attitudes underpinning the protocol itself. These protocols confront young people who are severely ill, causing them to reckon with the issue of procreation and banking gametes at the same time as they face their own mortality. This is especially challenging since the consent process requires them to designate a person who can use the gametes in case of their premature death or mental incapacity.

None of the extreme cases of parental 'interference' in white families (where parents were perceived as undermining the medico-legal notion of autonomy of a young person) were treated as a matter of culture. In one instance, a young man in his thirties said that he had felt devastated when he found out that his father had deprived him of the opportunity of sperm banking, by foreclosing any discussion on fertility prior to his treatment at sixteen. The other, described by a specialist nurse (FPR9), was a case of a young man who was 'coerced' by his mother to undergo fertility analysis following treatment, even though he was not emotionally ready to know or deal with the outcome of the test. She said:

> Yeah, she was sort of trying to persuade him ... to go ahead for it and that's what concerned us and, you know, we were sort of a little bit uncomfortable with that, really. Cos yes, he was sixteen, but, you know, he didn't need to know at that point in time, but she was certainly encouraging him and pushing him along that line.

Since follow-up consultations can involve potentially embarrassing discussions about sexuality, fertility and contraception, some specialist nurses felt that young people over sixteen must exercise their medico-legal right to autonomy. Interestingly, white parents wishing to accompany their children over sixteen for a consultation was recognised as an emotional issue of 'not being able to let go'. However, such 'intrusion' by South Asian parents was often treated suspiciously as representing a paternalistic family culture.[3] At the same time, while encouraging the autonomy of young people in clinical encounters, a desire for confidentiality by patients of South Asian origin is mysteriously transformed into secrecy, as we see later. It seems that the 'visibility of difference' of certain patients, and wider generalisations about their culture, interrupts the sensitivity and communicative reflexivity underpinning the notion of cultural competence, as explained below.

Of Sperm Banking, 'Asian' Men, and the Taboo on Masturbation

In some of the more reflective accounts professionals suggested that, when faced with patients and families of South Asian background, they were not sure to what extent what they observed reflected culture, religion or simply issues of gender or age. This, however, is a communicative strategy for marking minorities as the 'distant other' rather than closer to themselves. For instance, sperm banking and semen analysis are very emotive subjects for young men for the reasons discussed above. It is not hard to imagine the emotional, physical and social embarrassment of having to 'produce a sample' within an impersonal, public space at a time when a young man is already dealing with a life-threatening illness; especially if little psychological support is offered regarding what to expect during the process (see Chapple et al. 2007) or its long-term implications.

Clinicians across oncology and reproductive medicine recognised the complex interplay of serious illness, gender and age, and would try to offer young men the choice of discussing the subject with a male member of staff. For example, FPR9 acknowledged the emotional issues enmeshing fertility analysis for young men, and advised them to postpone having a test until they 'needed to know'. However, she somehow felt unsure about the religious/cultural issues when dealing with young men of South Asian origin:

> [T]here is definitely sensitivity about semen analysis discussions, with the South Asian men ... one of my difficulties is knowing about the cultural issues that affect that ... is it right to talk to them about this, and I always ask their permission first: 'I would like to talk to you about this, is that OK?' But it's sort of knowing, are they just saying that 'cos they've known me for a long time and, and yes they

> feel comfortable with me, or is there a cultural thing where they actually shouldn't really be talking about ...

In response to the Interviewer suggesting that it might just be a gender issue:

> Yes, might be a gender thing, male to female. So I'm not sure. I always approach it quite carefully and sensitively ... And each one I approach ... I always think, I'm going to offend somebody ... and fortunately I don't, or I don't appear to have [laughs].

Closely affiliated to the above was another popular story in the field, about the refusal of 'Asian' men to pursue sperm banking due to a religious proscription on masturbation (see Tomlinson and Pacey 2003; Ogle et al. 2008). South Asian, especially Muslim, men were perceived as having greater difficulties in 'producing a sample', and needing the advice or approval of a mullah (religious preacher versed in Islamic personal law). As PR12 remarked, 'And sometimes we have had some of our Asian boys refuse to store samples, because I think in some religions the masturbation ... is deemed as a sin, and so have actually refused'. The point being contested here is not that there might be Muslim men who choose to refuse the option of banking sperm, but rather how generalisations about religious groups are circulated within teams based on isolated instances reported by colleagues. Further, such generalisations reflected reified notions of religion perceived as determining men's ability to 'produce a sample' (FGD3 S2: 8). It was assumed that a 'lack of experience' leads to poor success rates and that, often, the men have to be accompanied by their wives (MPR2 S1; FGD 3). However, on further probing, some professionals did acknowledge that white patients were as likely to find the process emotionally or/and physically challenging, and might want their partner to accompany them.

Out of the sixteen men of South Asian origin who took part in the research, one knew before diagnosis that he was not fertile, and four had not been able to bank a sample (for entirely non-religious reasons). Two of these (of Pakistani origin) were Muslim, the third (of Indian origin) said that he was from a 'liberal Muslim' family with no prescriptions about what he could or could not do, and the fourth was from a Sikh family who did not follow any religion. Each had been seriously ill and in severe pain around the time of diagnosis. Only one Muslim man of Pakistani origin (not included above) said that he had declined sperm banking since he had two daughters and their family was complete.

While the act of masturbation in itself might be considered *haram* (unlawful) within dominant interpretations across Sunni and Shia Islam, it was considered lawful by the Muslim participants in this research within the therapeutic context of a life-threatening illness (also see Inhorn 2007a). One of the men (of Bangladeshi origin), who was more engaged with religious law, suggested that the status of the act (masturbation) is proximate to coitus interruptus, where the sperm is stored for later use by the couple. This, however, does not consider the conflicting interpretations of the practice of coitus interruptus within Islamic cultures (Chattoo 1990). Rather it reiterates the innovative modes of engaging with global 'scapes' of technology and ideas introduced by ARTs (Appadurai 1996). One of the specialists in reproductive medicine, a Muslim himself, dismissed these concerns about masturbation and banking as being misguided cultural representations of those who do not understand Islam (such as, 'people of African origin'). Indeed, most participants had, retrospectively, reconciled themselves to the issue within the therapeutic context, relying on their own interpretation, lived knowledge or misgivings about the use of IVF as being 'unnatural'. Only a couple of men had sought advice from a religious mentor or a *maulvi*. As pointed out by one of the men, he did not need to consult a *maulvi* since he was a devout Muslim and knew right from wrong. These plural engagements with religion remind us, yet again, about the role of biographical context and limitations of a 'community approach' in matters of faith and the use of ARTs.[4]

Of Conjugality, Arranged Marriages and Absence of Romantic Love

It is important to mention that the process of consent for storage of gametes (eggs/embryos/sperm) often redefines casual, transitory sexual relationships as quasi-conjugal ones, forcing couples as young as 16 to 19 years of age to think about commitment to each other and the possibility of wanting to have children together. Hence, while younger people across ethnic groups might have been pursuing the ideal type of a 'pure relationship' premised on a notion of choice, love and trust (Giddens 1991), they were drawn back within the fold of a dominant script of commitment and conjugality tied to 'reproductive intent' and parenting (Turney 2011). Needless to say, some relationships survived the test of loyalty and commitment, irrespective of age, while others crumbled under the pressure.

For example, one of the professionals (FGD3) mentioned the case of a white man whose fertility was affected by treatment, though he already had a child from a previous relationship. He broke off a long-term relationship with his partner under pressure, when she insisted on having a child using donor insemination. Neither her desire to have a child using a donor nor his inability to 'get his head round' donor insemination were attributed to pro-natalism or resistance to the idea of donor insemination in the wider culture (Haimes 1993). As observed by others, infertility in men is associated with greater stigma and secrecy in most cultures due to its close association with impotency, emasculation, and notions of descent and legacy (Haimes 1993; Carmeli and Birenbaum-Carmeli 2000; Bharadwaj 2003; Inhorn 2004; Simpson 2004a).

In contrast, during the same discussion (FGD3), the example of an 'Asian' man who refused to let his wife use preserved embryos from a previous relationship (prior to starting treatment) was easily attributed to 'both personal and cultural' reasons, as reflected in the following comment of a senior oncology nurse:

> And I think that is one of the things that some of our patients who have married and have had failed relationships is possibly... (due to) lack of libido, early menopause is quite hard for some ... And particularly if it's been ... an arranged marriage, like I said, that they haven't had the background knowledge of what the person has been through, because that is sometimes not shared and discussed as much. (FPR12)

As suggested earlier, within this stereotyped view of Asian/arranged marriages, conjugality is defined in terms of reproduction and perceived as being mutually exclusive of romantic love. This naive view betrays ignorance of how such matches and romantic relationships are negotiated by the young people within South Asian families (see Mody 2008). A wider conflation between arranged and forced marriages thus helps to redraw the boundaries between self and immigrant-settler as the distant other (Ahmad 2006), despite the familiarity with difference introduced through the notion of culturally competent care. I want to take this process of othering a bit further, and explain how a preconceived notion of a seamless relationship between (South Asian) individual and community culminates in a notion of 'a culture of secrecy and deceit'.

A Culture of Secrecy and Deceit?

It is quite intriguing how a request for confidentiality, a privilege of any patient within the NHS, was construed as a desire for 'secrecy' within 'Asian' families who were not willing to share intimate details about use of NRTs with members of their extended family. (The logistics of living within a complex/extended household might make privacy more of an issue for some.) According to an oncology nurse:

> [T]hey seemed to want more confidentiality with families ... I've certainly had a number who don't want their families to know anything about them if they're going for fertility assessment. So that was something that they'd decided they wanted to do, but it was very much their decision rather than their family's decision. Whereas with the British girls, you know... and males, they didn't mind the families being involved.

Why is the assertion of a right to privacy (in contrast with the image of the patriarchal family undermining this right) seen as problematic here? Needless to say, couples from white backgrounds do not disclose such intimate details of treatment to everybody within *their* extended family. The underlying assumption here is that South Asian families and communities operate as a seamless moral unit without boundaries between self and significant others (see Chattoo and Ahmad 2008 on the notion of relational autonomy). The sub-theme of privacy/secrecy, however, quickly transformed into one of a 'culture of silence' and even deceit. Note how an individual's ethical transgression signals the presence of collective attitudes within a culture or community in the following excerpt (not related to cancer):

> [A] lot [of South Asian Muslims] say they cannot have sperm unless they're married to the person who produced the sperm, so really sperm donation is out. So we have had couples coming through who bring in a brother but then they don't want their wife to know, and we will not do it then. Know what I mean, and there's a lie, we're (not) colluding with sort of lies. (PR13)

I am not able to comment on the context and contradiction within this case (i.e. why a husband would lie to his wife when he himself was subverting the dominant norm on sperm donation) since I did not conduct this interview myself. Nor can I estimate how often these requests might be made (although see Tremayne, this volume). However, the perception of 'Asians' as 'deceitful' resurfaced again when some professionals working within reproductive medicine (across two sites) talked about secrecy surrounding donor conception: 'It's going to be a tightly held secret within the family; they are not going to tell the child'. As we know, a majority of white couples prefer donor anonymity and secrecy about their children having been donor conceived. Despite a recent change (Department of Health 2010) to the UK Human Fertilisation and Embryology Act 2008, withdrawing donor anonymity, it is still not mandatory for parents to disclose this information to the child, despite her/his legal entitlement to disclosure at the age of 18. Indeed, desire for secrecy has been cited as one of the reasons for couples or individuals to seek a donor overseas (Pennings 2002; Blyth, Frith and Farrand 2005; Culley et al. 2011).

Revisiting the Practice of Cultural Competence

One of the major dilemmas posed by the rhetoric on cultural competence in health care within the British context is a reconciliation of policy focus on cultural and religious difference (with a view to providing more equitable care) with that on individual choice. This, paradoxically, results in bureaucratic responses to 'diversity management' and 'training', which, I argue, reinforces essentialised perceptions of minoritised cultures as static and homogenous wholes, reproduced through individuals across generations. Health professionals expect to have standardised guidelines that can tell them about health or religious beliefs of a 'Muslim', an 'Asian' or an 'African-Caribbean' patient or carer. Such a view, however, undermines the neo-liberal focus within policy on greater individual choice and the new rhetoric of 'no decision about me without me' (Department of Health 2006, 2009). The insecurity posed by assumptions about other cultures interrupts communication and prevents the professionals from asking basic questions related to choice, as reflected in the extract below:

> [S]o I would like that guidance, specifically about the males really … and what they are allowed to do and what they're not allowed to do and what, what we need to be sensitive about … and their ability to provide specimens, obviously, that's the main thing, and whether it is OK to talk to them about it. (FPR6, my emphasis)

As suggested earlier, health-related choices made by individuals from minoritised cultures and religions are assumed to reflect coercive imperatives undermining choice. Here, the binary between culture and individual choice helps to reconstitute the 'immigrant-settler'. In contrast, the decisions made by individuals from the white majority ethnic group are perceived as reflecting modernity and choice – rendering invisible the presence of culture in their decisions as well as the similarities across and differences within groups (especially white minorities that are less visible).

It is important to acknowledge that these dominant perceptions about minority ethnic cultures are often reinforced by attempts of those designated as community leaders (typically men) at reconstituting an 'imagined' moral community (Anderson 1991) premised on difference. Culture is reified as a thing with fixed attributes of a unique 'community', accompanied by a public display of unity and solidarity, mobilised for political purposes in an attempt at making claims to substantive citizenship rights (Knott 1991). Hence, such claims might reflect a subversive practice or moment in relation to exclusionary practices within wider society (Baumann 1997: 239). However, as mentioned earlier, demotic voices contest and discredit the notion of a homogenous community and culture, reflecting a reality of communities within community and cultures within community that are contextually negotiated and defined. In practice, far from being a unity, culture and community are dialogic sites of subjectivity, marked by constant moral debate and conflict over right and wrong within and between generations, undergoing change over time.

We need to deconstruct this twin process of essentialisation to facilitate reflexivity, enabling professionals to respond to the needs of people from minority ethnic groups without recourse to generalisations. This is especially important since professional assumptions and judgements about the needs of people from minority ethnic groups have a bearing on patterns of referrals to health and social care support. Muslim women, for example, may not be offered prenatal tests for genetic conditions since it is assumed that they will not be willing to terminate a pregnancy (see Atkin and Anionwu 2010). Religion, as a collective body of beliefs and practices, only provides moral boundaries for choices related to the use of medical technologies within a particular biographical context. It does not predefine individual negotiations of such moral choices (Shaw 2000; Remennick 2006; Atkin et al. 2008) or the extent to which these boundaries might be pushed and redefined at a collective level, at different historical points in time (Inhorn and Birenbaum-Carmeli 2008).

I want to end with a long excerpt from the account of an oncology nurse specialist to illustrate how professionals negotiate the emotional complexities of the lives of individuals they are caring for. It is interesting how a constant reminder of difference by the interviewer (not myself) reinstates uncertainty about culturally competent practice, even though she provides a very sensitive account of the complexity of intersectionality between gender, religion and personal belief. The extract relates to her interpretation of the situation of a young woman from a family of Pakistani Muslim background, who refused to have a hysterectomy when her cancer had spread. Everybody else in the team had assumed that the reason was religious and partly to do with pressures of an arranged marriage. The reader might notice that this is the iconic case of the patriarchal 'Asian' family perceived as preventing their unmarried daughter from having treatment.

> Nurse Specialist (NS): I've got a young lady at the moment, an Asian lady ... she'd had chemotherapy and knew that the chemotherapy it would make her infertile, but then refused to have the hysterectomy ... there were lots of questions around it, about whether or not it was because of religious reasons or whether or not it was because she definitely wanted to have children ... And so she gave lots of different reasons for it, depending on which particular person was trying to persuade her to have the hysterectomy. Because there was a point where she was potentially going to bleed to death, but it was resolved, and she said, 'No, I'd rather die than have the hysterectomy'.
>
> Interviewer: So what would have been the religious reasons for refusing a hysterectomy that she put forward?
>
> NS: She had (religious) leaders who came in and spoke to her about it. I think it [assumption about her refusal] was to do with arranged marriages, generally ... But then, when I spoke to her, it wasn't [so]. The impression she gave to me was it wasn't about necessarily religious grounds. It was more about who she saw herself as a person, and that without her womb ... she couldn't have children, then she wasn't who she perceived herself to be. And that was where I went with her really and had to take it on that value.
>
> Interviewer: How was it handled by the professionals?

NS: [Sighs] I think it was hard for other professionals, particularly when it was felt to be due to religious reasons ... There was a couple of the medical staff who followed her belief who spoke to her about it as well ... it felt to me, this great big [thing], who could try and make her change her mind ... I didn't feel that that was appropriate for her, 'cos she clearly understood the implications of her decision and, and there were clearly very many different levels to the decision that she'd made ... But the medical staff felt that because she was an Asian girl and because of her Muslim religion then this was all related to that really, and, and I don't feel [they] recognised her as an individual.

Interviewer: And when you say the medical staff found it more difficult ... do you mean that other nursing staff didn't find it as difficult, or were other nurses not as involved?

NS: Other nurses weren't as involved 'cos a lot of these conversations were happening in outpatients ... but it came up in lots of meetings and, and I [questioned myself] is it me? 'Should I be pushing this person more and should I be trying to persuade her more? And should I be killing myself as everyone else is, or feeling frustrated with her for this decision that she's made ... am I not being a professional and following this patient's best interests?' But no, and, and I still believe that was what she wanted and that was how she needed support.

Interviewer: ... and challenging.

NS: So you take that step back out of that box and go, hang on a minute, let's look at the whole picture and ... So yeah, because people question whether the family were bringing pressure on her ... I didn't, and I saw her on her own. I saw her with the family and I talked to them, and, and I think the family would have gone with whatever she'd wanted.

[Towards the end]

Interviewer: You know, sort of just thinking again about the South Asian population if there was anything you'd want to pull out?

NS: Not particularly ... I suppose, I treat everybody as an individual and, and I'm aware of their religious issues ... not 'issues', that's the wrong word. I don't treat the Muslim families any differently to how I treat the white population. I suppose my question from this is ... as to whether I'm wrong in that, and that's probably quite important to me now, because the questions you asked me, and certainly thinking through it, makes me question, 'Do I need to be dealing with them in a different way?

The Nurse Specialist in the above excerpt provides a good example of resisting the dominant, essentialist discourse on 'Asian' families by 'taking a step back' and treating the young woman as an individual, in an attempt to understand the choices she had made. She was willing to question her own response (given the interviewer's prompt to 'pull out differences'), especially in the face of a dilemma of duty of care towards her patient.

Concluding Comments

I suggested earlier that the social science community needs to reflect critically on how it might inadvertently reconstitute essentialist perceptions of minoritised ethnic communities by using analytical frameworks premised on dualisms: between majority and minority, immigrant and host, traditional and Western cultures. This involves an anti-essentialist conceptual shift in recognising difference as part of self rather than a defining feature of the other, as suggested by Carsten (2000) within the context of kinship studies. One way to make this shift, following Hall (1996) is to disassociate ethnicity from its anti-racist paradigm and use it in a positive sense of identities (and culture as language) that are both specific and responsive to dialogue and transformation (for a review, see Papastergiadis 1997). Such a move can help to challenge discrimination against people of minoritised cultures or cultural racism and yet seek equal citizenship rights for those who might, at one point, have been considered settlers or immigrants. We have to link in the policy and practice agenda of culturally competent care to what we have learnt from these debates within social sciences. A failure to recognise this link, as argued elsewhere (Chattoo and Atkin 2012), has meant that despite a focus on multiculturalism and anti-racist legislation in the UK, little progress has been made in actually dealing with racism, or in addressing prejudice and discrimination in health and welfare provision.

Notes

1. An 'abstract system' here is premised on expert knowledge that helps to deal with the threat of the uncertain, by regulating behaviour and codifying practice, thereby seeking to eliminate situations and experi-

ences that might otherwise require emotional or moral engagement at an individual level.

2. This research was supported by a grant from Cancer Research UK (CRUK) (C8351/A9005). My thanks to Karl Atkin (PI) and Marilyn Crawshaw for their contribution to the project, and to Rosie Tozer for her help with the professional focus group discussions and interviews. I would also like to thank all the participants who were generous with their time and support. The research was approved by the NHS National Research Ethics Service (07/H1307/181) and the Human Research Ethics and Governance Committee, University of York (Department of Health Sciences).
3. It would be interesting to draw comparisons with the legal and ethical controversy generated by the extreme case where Barry and Natasha Smith tried to negotiate access to their son's frozen sperm following his death, to fulfil their desire to be grandparents using a surrogate mother (see http://news.bbc.co.uk/1/hi/health/572377.stm, accessed 5 February 2012). While this seems like an attempt at transforming a 'bad' death into a 'good' death, following Simpson (2001b), drawing on a recognition of their 'right' to be grandparents, the request was denied on ethical and legal intricacies of consent, as well as the welfare of the child argument. The chairman of the Human Fertilisation and Embryology Authority (HFEA) was quoted as saying, 'We would all like to be grandparents. It doesn't mean we have the right to carry around the eggs and sperm of our children, looking for someone to bring them to life'. Needless to say, the potential use of ARTs creates new cultural solutions to issues of procreation, while the boundaries of the ethical debates over what is acceptable are constantly shifting and internally contested.
4. A comparative perspective is useful in understanding differences within and similarities across different ethnic and religious groups. For example, a shortage of gamete donors in South Asian communities in the UK (HFEA 2006) cannot simply be attributed to a religious or cultural proscription, since the demand for egg donors outweighs the number of donors. This implies different personal engagements of potential donors and recipients within the same community, as well as gendered responses to egg and semen donation (Hirsch 1999; Simpson 2004b; Purewal and van den Akker 2006; Hudson et al. 2009, see also this volume).

Sangeeta Chattoo is a visiting fellow in the Department of Health Sciences, University of York, UK. She is a social anthropologist by background and has carried out fieldwork in India and the UK. Her theoretical interests and publications engage with health as a site of subjectivity and the interrelations between self, community and state, with a special focus on marginalised communities. She is currently working on haemoglobinopathies as a case study of the interface between new genetics, ethnicity and citizenship within a globalising turn in public health. She has co-edited (with G. Craig, K. Atkin and R. Flynn) *Understanding 'Race' and Ethnicity: Theory, History, Policy, Practice* (2012), and is an editor for *Ethnicity and Health*.

Chapter 11

Knock, Knock, 'You're my Mummy'

Anonymity, Identification and Gamete Donation in British South Asian Communities

Nicky Hudson and Lorraine Culley

Involuntary childlessness is consistently described as a devastating life experience with implications for individuals and couples (Franklin 1997; Throsby 2004; Culley and Hudson 2009a). In many communities, infertility disrupts expected biographical trajectories and cultural scripts around becoming a parent (Letherby 1999; Becker 2000; Hudson 2008). In particular, the lack of continuation of familial connections and the chance to 'pass on' biogenetic relatedness, characterises the loss described by those who experience infertility (Becker 2000). For many of these individuals, assisted reproductive technologies (ARTs) such as IVF may be available to overcome infertility and achieve the culturally sanctioned transition to parenthood. However, in some cases, the nature of an individual's infertility means that their own biogenetic material, in the form of eggs or sperm, needs to be substituted (e.g. in the case of poor egg quality in women), or provided where none previously existed (as in the case of donor sperm for the treatment of single women or azoospermia in male partners). Under these circumstances a donor, or 'third party', can be used to supply the missing gametes (eggs or sperm).

Third-party assisted conception is a complex and often controversial 'treatment' for infertility given its potential for disrupting traditional familial relationships and networks (Blyth and Landau 2004). Fears about the 'risks' that third-party treatment may present to accepted categories of relatedness (mother, father, sibling, etc.) become visible through a discussion of their use (Edwards 1999, 2002; Hirsch 1999). Correspondingly, publics have expressed concerns about the 'limits' of such technologies in this context (Hirsch 1999) and tend to draw upon existing matrices of kin relations and idioms of kinship in order to describe and give meaning to what they see as the implications of ARTs (Strathern 1992b; Edwards 2002; Culley and Hudson 2009a). As such, ARTs have been used as a means to illuminate the problem of 'nature' and the contested binary between what we respectively come to know as the 'social' and the 'biological', particularly as they relate to the category of 'parent' (Strathern 1992a). However, wider discussion of the public perceptions of ARTs, and in particular of treatment involving donated gametes, remains relatively modest (Hudson et al. 2009). This absence persists despite the ongoing public debates about donation and the fact that currently in the UK approximately 11 per cent of all cycles of fertility treatment conducted involve the use of donor gametes (HFEA 2011a).

One aspect of donation that has received public attention in recent years is the issue of donor anonymity (HFEA 2011b). In the UK, the majority of donors are anonymous to the recipients of that donation at the point of treatment. However, since 2005, gamete donors are required by law to allow identifying information about them to be released to any future offspring should they request this information after the age of 18 (Department of Health 2004). Research suggests that there is no clear public consensus as to whether a particular kind of relationship between donors and recipients and their offspring is appropriate (Hudson et al. 2009). Debates about the impact this has had on donor recruitment continues in the UK (Purewal and van den Akker 2009; Hamilton 2010; Tomlinson et al. 2010) as demand for donor gametes continues to outstrip supply. More recently, donor shortages appear to be leading to an increase in the numbers of people travelling overseas in order to access treatment using donor gametes (Culley et al. 2011). Despite this context, little is known about how a wide range of publics understand and engage with ARTs. This is especially significant in that it is members of 'the public' who are required to engage with these technologies via the process of donation.

Ethnicity, Religion, ARTs and Donation

Infertility is a highly stigmatised condition in British South Asian communities, but there is also some evidence that treatment involving a third party is regarded as socially, and in some cases religiously, unacceptable (Culley et al. 2006a; Culley and Hudson 2007, 2009b; Purewal and van den Akker 2007, 2009; Simpson, Blell and Hampshire this volume). Correspondingly, the recruitment of gamete donors from minority ethnic communities has continued to be perceived as a particular challenge (HFEA 2005; Hudson et al. 2009; Purewal and van den Akker 2009), with treatment seekers from these communities especially disadvantaged in this respect (HFEA 2005; Kan et al. 1998; Golombok and Murray 1999). It has been suggested that this lack of minority ethnic donors may mean that treatment-seeking couples from these communities may be more likely to need to use a known or family donor, in the absence of so-called 'altruistic' donors recruited by clinics. However, little in-depth research has been conducted that interrogates the complex issue of willingness to donate gametes amongst members of minority ethnic communities in the UK. One small-scale study (eight women) suggests that South Asian women may be less likely than white women to donate their eggs due to socio-cultural norms within South Asian communities (Purewal and van den Akker 2009). In a related questionnaire study, the authors suggest that 'Asian' women are less likely to consider donating their eggs than 'Caucasian' women due to 'wider cultural differences' including increased religiosity (Purewal and van den Akker 2006). Our own study of public perceptions of gamete donation in British South Asian communities[1] highlights several possible complexities around the acceptance of gamete donation generally, with its implications for kinship and familial connections, and the recruitment of donors (Culley et al. 2006a; Culley and Hudson 2007, 2009a). In this chapter we address the specific issue of donor anonymity and what 'knowing' the donor might mean for existing conceptualisations of relatedness, parenthood and community within British South Asian communities. In doing so we add to what is currently known about donor motivations in relation to the impact of the removal of donor anonymity in the UK. Crucially, the chapter focuses on what implications these understandings might have for the recruitment of donors and the use of 'family' or 'known' donors from within these minority communities.

The GAMDON Study

The GAMDON study builds on previous work on infertility with British South Asian communities carried out by the authors (Culley et al. 2004, 2006a, 2006b) but was particularly concerned to explore issues around donation more fully within these communities. The study was based on a qualitative interpretive design using focus groups as the primary data collection method.

Fourteen single-sex focus groups with a total of 100 participants of Indian, Pakistani and Bangladeshi origin were conducted in three English cities. Ten of the groups were with women (n=63) and four with men (n=37). A range of age groups were represented in the study. Five of the groups were conducted by trained community facilitators in South Asian languages (two in Punjabi, two in Bengali [Sylheti dialect] and one in Urdu), and nine groups were conducted in English by the authors.

Significantly, none of the participants were recruited on the basis of their own fertility histories or on whether they had ever acted as donors themselves. Rather, the study more generally and the focus groups in particular were designed to elicit the participants' views on the 'community' discourses surrounding gamete donation. This method, which we had used previously (Culley, Hudson and Rapport 2007), is designed to explore a potentially 'sensitive' topic, by depersonalising it for the focus group members. Vignettes were used in order to give people some information about gamete donation, to depersonalise the issue, and to generate discussion through a consideration of the stories. We found this approach effective in eliciting what Cunningham-Burley, Kerr and Pavis (2001) refer to in their similar work on new genetics as 'lay expertise' (ibid.: 8). The participants were asked about the importance of children, attitudes to fertility treatment and in particular how they felt people in their own communities would respond to a number of issues concerning the use of donated eggs and sperm, and their willingness to act as donors of eggs and sperm.[2] The groups in English were tape recorded and transcribed in full. The groups in South Asian languages were tape recorded, translated and transcribed into English by the facilitator who conducted the group. Framework analysis was used in order to develop the themes and theoretical insights from the data (Ritchie and Spencer 1994).

Findings from this study, which relate to views of donation more generally, are reported elsewhere (Culley et al. 2006a; Culley and Hudson 2007, 2009a). Here we discuss the responses of participants to the issue of donor anonymity, with the emphasis on the impact of identifiable donation on both the potential gamete donor and on donation rates. The findings are organised around a discussion of: the general acceptability of gamete donation as a treatment; the impact of gender, culture and religion on views of donor anonymity; and finally a consideration of the use of 'known' donors in fertility treatment.

The Acceptability of Gamete Donation as a Treatment 'Option'

In general, participants felt that the use of third-party assisted conception would be very much a treatment of last resort for South Asian couples. Most participants felt that while infertility is highly stigmatised, treatment using donated gametes would be regarded as socially and culturally unacceptable in most South Asian families. However, given the suffering of childless couples, many participants felt that such treatment should be available, and that despite a general social disapproval, some couples would wish to undertake treatment using donor gametes. This varied somewhat according to the specific community in question. As will be seen later, many of the Muslim participants in particular expressed concerns about the religious acceptability of donating and using donated gametes.

However, the general attitude to gamete donors was favourable, and several participants praised what they saw as a highly commendable and altruistic act, which would help to alleviate the suffering of infertile couples in a context where infertility was highly problematic: 'It is very, very admirable and, you know, you're talking about it and discussing it makes me think about all those women who do, have done it for other people and that, that, I take my hat off' (Indian Hindu and Sikh women, FG5). However, positive views of donation tended to be expressed prior to the participants being given information about the removal of donor anonymity.[3] When the issue of the removal of donor anonymity was raised by the group facilitator, their concerns about this were clear. The next three themes to be presented here discuss these specific concerns in more detail, particularly as they relate to 'knowing' the donor.

Gendered Concerns: The Emotional Impact on Female Donors and the Financial Impact on Male Donors

When discussing the removal of donor anonymity, all of the female groups spontaneously began to discuss the issue of a female donor meeting the donor-conceived child. The majority of women regarded such a possibility as highly problematic. Most discussed this in relation to how they would feel in this situation, and the most common view was that this would bring emotional turmoil to their lives in the future. This appeared to be less of a concern for the men, and prompting was required to elicit men's views on the specific issue of a donor meeting 'their' child later in life.

Many of the women in the study had concerns about becoming donors themselves in this context. This appeared to be due to the permanence of the emotional risk involved, and that a woman would 'always wonder' about the outcome of the donation. The common idiom of a child 'turning up' was used again and again by the women, related to the fear of meeting the child unexpectedly in the future: 'I was considering it a few years back but I always got scared that someone's gonna knock on my door in twenty years' time and say 'Oh, you're my biological mother' [laughter] (Indian and Sikh women, FG5). 'Knock, knock, you're my mummy' [laughter] (Indian Hindu women, FG12).

The idea that a donor-conceived adult would seek out their donor in the future was a highly contentious issue. Anxiety and emotions would run high if such a person wanted to meet, due to the fact that some of the women felt they would not be able to disentangle themselves from the emotions involved in donating biological material that would become (or, for some, was already) a child: 'I suppose it wouldn't be your child as such once you've donated it. See, really, I think, it's my child but it isn't, so I think that's the hardest bit – is it or isn't it? I don't know, I think that's what, that would be a bigger step' (Indian Hindu and Sikh women, FG9).

The idea that this would not be as difficult a decision for men was discussed in the groups and the men reported far fewer concerns than the women about meeting any subsequent children. Some men reported being happy to meet a future child, so long as there was no ongoing commitment to that child: 'Why not? One hundred per cent I would like to meet the child, not for bringing him home, but only just to see him' (Indian Sikh man, FG7). 'I will not make any extra effort to travel 1,000 km to see him, but if I see him in any party or elsewhere I don't mind meeting him' (Pakistani Muslim man, FG10).

There appeared to be much less concern from the men with regard to emotional consequences of meeting a person conceived from their donation, who was viewed almost as a distant relative. However, a small number of men raised concerns about potential economic consequences of donation, such as financial responsibilities for offspring and the potential implications for inheritance: 'I have only one concern, that one day he may come and ask for his share in my inheritance' (Pakistani Muslim man, FG10). The issue of financial inheritance is highly significant in Islam, and a small number of Muslim women in one of the groups also raised the importance of a child's 'right to know' their biological father in Islamic teachings, bringing with it some concerns about ensuing financial obligations for the men. The impact of religion on decisions to donate is discussed more generally in the next section.

A number of studies have found differences between the ways in which men and women perceive the donation of gametes (Lessor et al. 1990; Bolton et al. 1991; Baluch, Fallone and Khan 1994; Kazem et al. 1995; Westlander et al. 1998; Kailasam, Sykes and Jenkins 2001; Urdapilleta, Chillik and Fernandez 2001; Chliaoutakis, Koukouli and Papadakaki 2002; Skoog-Svanberg et al. 2003; Isikoglu et al. 2006; Purewal and van den Akker 2006, 2009; Brett et al. 2008; Culley and Hudson 2009b), but are inconclusive with regards to precisely how gender may impact on decision making. In addition, few studies have explored this specifically in relation to the removal of donor anonymity. Our findings suggest that gender is an important factor in considering how donors may feel about being identified by donor-conceived children in the future, with more concerns about the potential for a child 'turning up' being expressed by the women (Purewal and van den Akker 2006). Participants in this study took the view that women would remain emotionally connected to the donated material and therefore saw donation as an emotionally risky act for women. Women were seen as inherently and essentially connected to parenthood through their emotional and embodied selves (Culley and Hudson 2009a). This would to some extent be negated in the case of anonymous donation, where the woman could be guaranteed never to meet the child, and therefore these 'maternal' feelings would potentially never be fully realised. Both male and female participants felt that men would not find this aspect of donation so problematic.

It was suggested that men did not perceive a genetically related donor-conceived child to be connected to them in any emotionally meaningful way (Culley and Hudson 2009a), identifying them only as 'causal' (biological) fathers, and not 'moral' (social) fathers (Draper and Ives 2009). However, alternative concerns about donor anonymity were considered by some of the male participants. In particular, the possibility was raised by some of the Muslim men that a person conceived using their sperm might later lay claim to an 'inheritance'. Although not a prominent theme in the discussions, the idea that a donor-conceived person could claim financial inheritance from his or her biological father is an important point. In the case of adoption more generally (to which the case of donation is often likened), within Islam 'official' adoption in the Western sense is not permitted: a child must keep his or her biological father's name and is entitled to a share of the family inheritance. If this model is mobilised in the case of gamete donation then a donor-conceived individual has a right to know his or her father and in turn to lay financial claim to that man's financial assets.

The Religious, Social and Cultural Context of Non-Anonymous Donation

The fact that identifiable donation could involve the potentially 'public' event of a donor-conceived person 'turning up' as an adult, meant that the act of donation would not only have implications for the individual donor, but also, importantly, for family and community members, as it would be difficult for the donor to conceal it from them. This had further implications for potential donors: even if they themselves were keen to donate, the social implications of this act may prevent them from doing so. This was especially the case for a younger, unmarried woman, who it was imagined would be the most likely to act in this capacity. The implications for her in the future were clearly of concern. This additional set of social or 'community-based' risks were discussed by both male and female participants. It was felt that there would be a particular set of consequences, especially for the conjugal relationship, either to future marriage prospects or for the stability of the relationship for those already married. Once again though, it was the women who were more likely to articulate fears about the consequences of a child 'turning up' in this context: 'So if you went and became a donor, and you did not tell anything ... you'd have forgot all about it, you did this, right? ...and you get married one day, someone comes knocking on your door, then do you tell your husband or what do you do?' (Pakistani Muslim woman, FG14).

The view that there would be consequences for a donor, if it were later revealed that they had acted in this role, was not restricted to the marital relationship. It was also felt by participants that the wider community would have 'something to say' on the matter and that this would be a cause for social concern more widely. As these Indian Muslim women discuss (FG11):

> A: Because our generation are moving with the times, but it's always gonna be the stigma attached to what the general community are gonna have to say about it.
>
> B: It's just not worth the hassle, is it?

Even if an individual were willing to act as a donor, and were willing to consider the possibility of a child wanting to meet them later in life, the potential disruption to their life that this might entail was considered too great a cost to a person's existing kinship networks.

The culmination of these discussions about the perceived risks of the donation process, especially for identifiable donors, was felt to be a decline in numbers of those willing to donate. When asked what might assist in increasing donation from South Asian communities, initially participants suggested that increased publicity and education amongst community members was needed to alert people to the need for donors. However, once the issue of the removal of donor anonymity was raised, it was felt that this introduced a further set of considerations into this process, making the recruitment of donors more difficult than simply 'raising awareness'. Participants felt that the personal cost to donors, in the context of South Asian kinship networks, may be too high for people to consider acting as a so-called 'altruistic' donor.

> I think for a lot of your donors, the thing that's gonna attract them to it is, as you say, the complete anonymity, and the fact that there is not gonna be any comeback. They've washed their hands of it; they've done their bit, washed their hands of it and they don't want to know. (Indian and Pakistani Muslim women, FG8)

An extensive debate continues in the UK about whether or not the removal of anonymity has led to a reduction in donors (Purewal and van den Akker 2009; Hamilton 2010; Tomlinson et al. 2010) and about the ways in which the numbers of donors could be improved. In common with earlier study findings, this research demonstrates explicit public concerns about the removal of anonymity for donors (Purdie et al. 1994; Lui and Weaver 1996; Westlander et al. 1998; Chliaoutakis, Koukouli and Papadakaki 2002). However, for the men and women in this study, there were perhaps added culturally specific concerns about an imagined 'community' response to the act of donation (Anderson 1991; Simpson 2000).

Donation, Islam and the Identification of Biological Origins

As we have described, religious ideas and practices were significant in shaping group discussions. In the groups with Muslim respondents, the discussions were primarily, but not exclusively, framed within the context of an understanding of Islamic teaching. For Muslim women and men, new reproductive technologies are framed within a discourse of risk that is primarily interpreted though their existing value and belief systems in which Islam plays a key role (Inhorn 2005; Clarke 2006, 2009). While there was some doubt and debate concerning the acceptability of gamete donation within Islam, many participants raised a series of objections to the practice that were derived from religious and cultural understandings.[4] This was particularly evident in the female groups and in relation to using donated sperm. Many of the Muslim women were well informed about religious teachings on the significance of the marital bond and the importance of the genetic connection of father and child in Islam. In this context women felt that it was unlikely that a Muslim couple would accept third-party assisted conception, at least using an anonymous sperm donor. Islam mandates biological inheritance: preserving the '*nasab*' or known biological origins of a child is a moral imperative, and third-party donation is seen to confuse issues of kinship, descent and inheritance, and thus effectively destroy a child's lineage. Sperm donation is therefore regarded as *zina* (adultery) (Inhorn 2005), and a child born by forbidden methods is a *laqith* (illegitimate).

There was less clarity about the religious acceptability of egg donation, and some of the Muslim women said that they would consider acting as a donor for family or close friends, to relieve the suffering of infertile women (see below). Several participants felt that decisions about using or donating gametes would require guidance from local religious scholars (imams). Within the Sunni tradition of Islam (predominant in the UK), several authoritative religious proclamations (*fatwas*) by esteemed religious scholars exist in relation to gamete donation. While artificial insemination with the husband's semen and IVF using the couple's own gametes are allowed, and the resulting child is the legal offspring of the couple, the use of a third party is strictly prohibited.

Religious discourses were remarkable by their absence in the discussions with the Hindu and Sikh participants. In these groups, talk about the acceptability of the donation and use of gametes was inflected by and articulated through a sense of South Asian culture or 'communal' identification, but this was not shaped by religious doctrine or teachings. Although the Hindu and Sikh groups shared the view that sperm donation was more problematic than egg donation, this was described as an artefact of South Asian 'culture' in which male lineage is seen to be most significant in kinship terms and therefore must be preserved (Culley and Hudson 2009a).

(A) I think a genetic link with the man is more...
(B) ...acceptable
(A) ...it's more acceptable in the community.
(I) Right. Why is that?
(C) Because of the sexism between, I think.
(D) I think because at the end of the day it is still a sperm that's coming from ... the male of the household; it's not something that's coming from outside.

(Indian Hindu and Sikh women, FG 5)

Therefore, whilst the perception of the risks associated with sperm donation were similarly discussed across the groups, they were interpreted within different frameworks of understanding:

'religion' for the Muslim groups, and 'culture' for the Sikh and Hindu groups.

Given the importance of preserving a child's genetic origins within both frameworks, having an unknown donor may be highly problematic, particularly for some Muslim couples. One solution to this dilemma that was discussed in the groups was the possibility of having a 'known' donor, usually in the form of a family member, who would preserve a bio-genetic link to the resulting child.

Family or 'Biogenetic' Donation

Although there were some concerns expressed about donation generally, donation within the family was seen as a comparatively risk-free option for recipient couples, at least in some scenarios. This was related in the discussions to the practice of 'informal adoption', which has historically served as a solution to infertility within communities in South Asia (Unisa 1999). All of the groups raised the issue of informal adoption spontaneously, and many participants knew or had heard of someone who had experience of this practice. In most cases of informal adoption a decision is made within the family that one son and his wife, who already have children, would 'give' their next child to the childless son and his wife. Although the extent of this practice is somewhat anecdotal here, the degree to which this practice was mentioned warrants further research in the UK setting. This traditional 'solution' to childlessness in South Asian communities meant that although the child was brought up by different parents, he or she was still closely related to the 'birth' couple and would remain within the immediate kinship network. Experience of this alternative form of reproduction and parenting allowed participants in all groups to explore the complexities involved with relatedness within families, as well as the risks related to 'secrets' within the family.

In comparison to unknown 'anonymous' donation, known donation (to a family member) was viewed as a relatively acceptable thing to do. For the female participants especially, the possibility of donating eggs anonymously was considered to be emotionally risky since there would always be a 'connection' to any child conceived from those eggs. This connection would not be reciprocated in an anonymous donation, however, with the donor being unable to locate or have a relationship with the child, and this would lead to emotional insecurity for the donor. This situation was not seen by the female participants as being solved by the removal of donor anonymity. In the case of a previously unknown donor child 'turning up' in eighteen years' time, this was perceived as being as problematic as anonymous donation, since the child would be an unknown entity and would therefore be emotionally and relationally 'risky'. However, by contrast, donating to a family member was considered acceptable, and even preferable, by some female participants. This may be related to the symbolic and cultural value placed on children in South Asian communities (Culley et al. 2004; Purewal and van den Akker 2007; Hudson 2008; Simpson 2013) in that relinquishing gametes to 'unknown' families or communities may equate to relinquishing related children to other kinship groups. This may serve to restrict the flow of donor gametes out of the family into unknown reproductive contexts. Known donation, by contrast, serves to maintain familial and emotional links with the donation and the subsequent child, as in informal adoption: 'It's not as if they're going to be separated from those children' (Pakistani Muslim woman, FG8).

However, this is not to say that donation within families was not considered to be contentious. Drawing on knowledge about informal adoption, an associated set of risks was discussed. For example, the perception was that family donors would want to intervene if they felt that 'their' child was not being cared for appropriately. This was matched by a corresponding fear on the part of the receiving couple, which related to concerns that a family donor would interfere and may ultimately wish to 'claim' the child: 'Oh by the way, can I have my baby please?' (Pakistani Muslim woman, FG8). These problems were seen as inevitably leading to family conflict and breakdown, with potential problems for the donor-conceived child or adult in future: 'I think that would quite create a lot of problems within the family' (Mixed female group, FG14).

These findings are similar to those reported in the existing literature on 'known' donation. For example, research with known donors suggests that they may prefer minimal or no contact with the donor offspring (see Purewal and van den Akker 2009). Baetens et al. (2000) found that known donors did feel a responsibility towards the child and hoped that they would be well cared for by the recipient couple. However, for Muslim couples there may be added considerations when choosing a 'family' donor. Although this 'solution' to infertility may negate the problem of the lack of a biogenetic connection, under Islamic law 'known' donation would still transgress the strict moral obligation for reproduction to take place only within heterosexual marriage (Inhorn 2005).

Conclusions

Gender, culture and religion are salient factors in understanding the impact of the removal of donor anonymity in the UK. For the Muslim groups in our study, Islam became the most important lens through which to view the process of donation, whilst Hindu and Sikh participants identified South Asian 'culture' as the defining feature of this discourse. However, across all groups, the gendered features of these articulations and understandings were clear, as were the different consequences for men and women. These examples highlight the complexity of understandings of gamete donation and the need to be mindful of a range of intersecting identifiers that may be important at different times and amongst different groups. The findings presented here confirm the importance of seeing public perceptions of ARTs as socially constructed and negotiated. As we have argued elsewhere however, it is important to avoid essentialising culture and to remain alert to the similarities in the experiences of majority and minority populations (Atkin 2004; Culley et al. 2006b; Hudson 2008; Culley and Hudson 2009b; see also Chattoo, this volume). Many of the concerns expressed about identifiable donation in our study, particularly those shaped by gender, can arise from people from all ethnic backgrounds. The complexity of conceiving using a third party represents an unsettling and disruptive set of dilemmas, regardless of ethnicity (Edwards 1999; Blyth and Landau 2004; Donovan 2006). As others have argued, gamete donation represents a challenge to received ideas of identity, and has implications for social reproduction that go well beyond the individual. For potential donors, it brings into play the creation of new and potentially disruptive and disturbing relationships, regardless of ethnicity (Edwards 1999; Donovan 2006).

However, avoiding culturally essentialist discourses does not mean denying that people are cultural beings, and there are examples in our work of the specific cultural locations that our participants occupied. Drawing on the historical example of informal, intra-family adoption allowed our participants to make sense of the process of known donation, for example. Although there were clearly benefits in having a genetically and emotionally linked donor, the participants were also able to articulate a particular set of risks associated with this arrangement, drawn from a shared tradition of intra-family adoption. Using this knowledge allowed participants to explore the potential disruption and emotional dilemmas that could be involved in known donation. This finding may have specific implications for the UK treatment context: if there continues to be a shortage of altruistic donors from minority ethnic communities, there may be more couples from these communities facing the dilemma of using a biogenetically related, family donor in order to achieve a pregnancy.

The gendering of the risks associated with donation was also culturally inflected. In our study it was felt by both male and female participants that gamete donation would be a more socially risk-laden process for women to engage in (especially for unmarried women), given their association in some contexts with constructions of 'family honour' (Inhorn 1994b). Participants felt that disclosure of the fact of donation, perhaps instigated by the 'turning up' of a donor-conceived person, could be highly detrimental to a donor's current and future conjugal and family relationships. It was felt that women are more vulnerable than men to social stigma and ostracism for apparently transgressing cultural norms in South Asian communities (Culley and Hudson 2009b). This particular articulation of a South Asian femininity 'at risk' through the process of donation was commonly discussed in the groups (ibid.), and was heightened in the context of identifiable donation.

A concern for, and empathy towards, infertile couples was very evident in this study. However, participants articulated concerns about donating eggs and sperm in general, and specifically in the context of identifiable donors. Our data demonstrate how culture, religion and gender may impact, in complex and intersecting ways, on attitudes to gamete donation.

Notes

1. 'Public Perceptions of Gamete Donation in British South Asian Communities'. Funded by the ESRC's Science in Society programme 2005–2006. Grant number: RES-160-25-0044.
2. Information about the process of donation and the law surrounding it was given to the participants during the course of the groups. The focus

groups were designed in this way to offer knowledge and understanding of the topic, as well as being data-collection 'events'.

3. The law on donor anonymity had recently changed at the time of data collection – a fact not widely known amongst participants.
4. It is also important to note, however, that there is a difference between official representations of religious ideas, and the experience of religion as 'lived'. It would be incorrect to assume that someone who identifies themselves as Muslim would not wish to consider using donated gametes in treatment, or donating gametes for the use of others. Religion may nevertheless play a significant role in decision making in relation to becoming a gamete donor.

Nicky Hudson is a Reader in Medical Sociology at De Montfort University, Leicester, and a sociologist with an interest in health, illness and medicine. She has particular expertise in social aspects of infertility and reproduction, and has completed a number of studies in this area funded by the Economic and Social Research Council, the Department of Health and local NHS trusts. She is currently engaged in a portfolio of work that explores the lived experience of chronic conditions such as endometriosis and asthma. Her PhD was a study of involuntary childlessness and the use of assisted reproductive technologies in British South Asian communities.

Lorraine Culley is emeritus professor of Social Science and Health at De Montfort University, Leicester. She is a sociologist by background and a graduate of the universities of Liverpool (BA, PhD) and London (MA). Her research is focused on social and political aspects of health and health care, with a particular emphasis on ethnic and gender inequalities, chronic conditions, social aspects of infertility, reproductive technologies and endometriosis. She has particular expertise in qualitative methodologies and in research that explores user perspectives of health and health care.

Chapter 12

Practitioner Perspective

Cultural Competence from Theory to Clinical Practice

Ana Liddie Navarro and Miriam Orcutt

As two junior doctors, both with bi-cultural backgrounds, who have trained and are now working in the UK, our interest in global health and medical anthropology has led us to volunteer and conduct research in several countries and health care settings. Bringing the perspectives and lessons we have learned back into our clinical practice in the UK has highlighted to us the importance of socio-cultural awareness. Here we reflect on the chapters by Chattoo, and Hudson and Culley, in conjunction with our own experiences in clinical practice, and consider what it means to deliver culturally competent practice.

Medical Practice and Socio-cultural Awareness

Health care professionals inevitably work within complex socio-cultural environments. In each interaction, doctors must balance a patient's ideas and expectations alongside their own. Through understanding the socially constructed nature of beliefs and actions, trust and ultimately patient care may be improved (American College of Obstetrics and Gynecologists 2011). In preparing health care professionals for the globalised medical workplace it is imperative for them to be 'culturally competent' in order to navigate effectively the complex and diverse socio-cultural worlds that come together in a clinical encounter. In what follows we outline the importance of socio-cultural awareness and competence, and consider some of the challenges that doctors might encounter when putting this theory into practice.

1. *The Dynamic Nature of Culture and the Patient–Doctor Relationship*

   Understanding cultural complexities, and their dynamic and contingent nature, can enable improvement in the efficacy of treatment and the relationship with the patient.

As highlighted by Chattoo, an individual's beliefs and priorities may change over time, as they interact with others in our increasingly multicultural and cosmopolitan society. Recent developments in anthropological thinking have moved away from a straightforward 'acculturation' model, whereby migrants and their children progressively adopt the cultural apparatus of their destination country in a linear fashion. The process of change is far more complex, contingent and dynamic, often resulting in completely new cultural forms and ways of being. We must therefore be careful to avoid generalisations about an individual's identity as defined by standard demographics, and consider the specific socio-cultural world they inhabit, seeing culture as one aspect of a fluid ethnic identity that may be constantly renegotiated and reconstructed (Barth 2000; Hampshire, Blell and Simpson 2012b). The temptation to make generalisations, and the problematic assumptions that may ensue, are illustrated by a recent encounter that one of us experienced.

> Case Study 1: During a local Obstetrics and Gynaecology placement while at school in England, one of us spent time in a fertility clinic. A 40-year-old lady from the Democratic Republic of Congo (DRC) attended with her husband for blood test results after many years of trying to have a child. She was told that the reason she had not been able to conceive was that she had already gone through menopause, which also meant, of course, that she would not be able to become pregnant in the future. Her reaction to this was a combination of anger and disbelief, alongside a feeling of injustice. There was an element of mistrust, as if we had the power to help but did not want to exercise this. She could not accept that she would never become pregnant, and declared that if she were in her own country this would be treatable.

> The consultation ended with her saying she was going back to DRC to see a doctor there. When the patient left the room, the doctor turned to me, shrugged his shoulders, and rationalised the encounter by explaining to me that 'some of these African cultures' place high reproductive demands on women. It is easy to make broad generalisations about the influence of culture on health care, but there is a very real danger of over-simplification. Of course there may well have been an element of culturally specific pressures and expectations around conception; but there were extra complexities here such as mistrust of another country's health care system, and possible communication barriers, as although the patient's English was deemed good enough not to need a translator, subtleties may have been missed.

Chattoo directs attention to the important question of how a more critical social science perspective can help to address this issue, at a time when 50 per cent of people of immigrant origin have been born in the UK. The increasing number of children born and brought up in families with mixed ethnic origins also renders simplistic categories meaningless. As the margins of our constructed categories begin to blur, methods for dealing with ethnicity in relation to culture must be flexible and respond to an individual's own identity and way of being, rather than a preformed stereotype.

2. *Decision Making: Balancing Autonomy, Capacity, Relationship and Kinship*

   Understanding patients' decision-making processes is imperative in order to facilitate informed health care choices.

Increased situational and cultural awareness is important at various stages of the health care consultation, including during the process of providing information, checking understanding, and appreciating the factors influencing a patient's decision making. In recent decades, the traditionally paternalistic role of doctors in the doctor–patient relationship has evolved into one that is more patient-centred, with patients' autonomy being central to practice. This places doctors in a key role as the providers of information and facilitators of informed decision making. This is done by assessing capacity: verifying that a patient understands the information relevant to that decision, can retain that information, and can use it to weigh up the choices and then communicate the decision back.

Whilst diagnoses and decisions may be perceived as clearly defined within an allopathic medico-social framework, other norms and values might influence a patient's understanding and perception of the treatment they are receiving. Operating within a framework that places high value on patient autonomy, health care professionals may find it difficult to recognise or understand decisions that appear to rely heavily on family and community, and in which a patient might not even factor their own wishes, or may find it difficult to disentangle their desires and priorities from those of a wider family network, for example. While health systems like the one in the UK are premised on an idea of individual autonomy and consent, this may sit unhappily with other social and moral frameworks that emphasise and prioritise connections and relations between people (Sariola and Simpson 2011). Managing the tensions that arise from this encounter can be a major challenge for health care professionals. On the one hand, even though autonomy is presumed it is important to recognise that an individual may choose to reject it. On the other hand, as Chattoo argues, it is always necessary to avoid assuming a 'seamless moral unit without boundaries between self and significant others'.

However, there are circumstances in which a health care professional has a duty of care, and it becomes important to identify points where collective decision making might tip into undue persuasion or coercion. Disentangling these can be challenging when differential power relations within families (based for example on gender, age/seniority or disability) come into play, and is particularly crucial when there is a minor, or an older person with cognitive impairment, or someone with learning disabilities involved. In each individual case, these situations must be handled with care, and the patient's best interests put foremost, with special consideration if the person has limited decision-making capacity (either because of age, learning disability, etc., or because their social circumstances limit their ability and authority to negotiate effectively).

3. *Recognising the Socially Constructed Nature of Health Care Professionals' own Practices and Values*

   With an appreciation of our own socio-cultural backgrounds and how these play into our assumptions and practice, we can better reflect on our influence on patient interactions.

A theme that is often understated in accounts of ethnicity and health care is the extent to which practitioners themselves also come with particular socio-cultural backgrounds and sets of experiences that play into their own assumptions and worldviews. In order to develop the most therapeutically helpful interventions in a socially diverse country such as the UK, it is important to develop ways of analysing professional reactions to otherness. An important element of this reaction is that health care professionals bring not only their own socio-cultural identities but also their background in allopathic medicine. As Chattoo explains, although health care professionals are governed by codes of professional conduct and ethics, in practice there is considerable ambiguity and variation. She also warns against projecting our own values and social constructions onto other people. During fieldwork in Zambia, one of us experienced some of these tensions first-hand:

> Case Study 2: Mrs Tembo was a 28-year-old woman with three children from a very remote village in Eastern Zambia. She came to me for a medical opinion, dehydrated and feverish with a fast heart rate and constant shortness of breath. She described heavy menstrual bleeding over the previous two months and appeared septic. I was concerned that she was dangerously ill, and urged her to visit the hospital immediately for a blood test, fluids and antibiotics. She told me that she could not leave her children and so would have to visit her parents first, who lived a four-hour walk away in the mountains of Malawi. She was struggling to walk even a couple of metres on flat ground and was not medically fit to make the journey. However, she could not be dissuaded and eventually it transpired that her husband was an alcoholic with two other wives whom she did not trust to be left alone with her children at home. She refused to leave the children with anyone else for fear of witchcraft, and in case they fell ill or died in her absence; if this happened she would be held responsible by her in-laws. She preferred to stay in the village with her children, even though she understood that she was very ill. I reiterated the seriousness of her situation. However, although I understood her decision within the context of constrained personal agency due to her social context and cultural beliefs, I did not realise until afterwards that in my reaction to it I was also projecting my own socially constructed beliefs of autonomy and agency onto the patient.

Challenges in Adopting a Culturally Competent Health Care Practice

Uncertainty and Subsequent Categorisation

There is a considerable body of evidence suggesting that health and social care professionals often fail to provide accessible and appropriate care to people from ethnic minority backgrounds (Scheppers et al. 2006; Zeh et al. 2014). As Hudson and Culley argue, it is of great importance to avoid essentialising culture and to remain alert to similarities in the experience of different minority and majority groups. One response to this challenge of embracing difference yet ensuring equality has been the development of the notion of 'cultural competence' skills among health care professionals (Leavitt 2002; Khanna, Cheyney and Engle 2009). Chattoo shows how an awareness of cultural difference can be a source of anxiety for health professionals. Although clinicians are professionally obliged to raise all possible treatment options, they may fail to do so because of presumed religious or cultural sensitivities, which, as Chattoo shows, can be a highly problematic scenario.

With regards to gamete donor anonymity, Hudson and Culley conclude that gender, culture and religion all play into patients' concerns and priorities in important ways, but the relative importance of these factors varies both within and between ethnic groups in complex ways. Whilst health care professionals may be acting out of goodwill, in their attempts to be culturally sensitive they may in fact end up being discriminatory in their actions. By trying to manage uncertainty when dealing with people of diverse social and cultural backgrounds, health care professionals may tend to categorise at the earliest opportunity. Indeed, pattern recognition is a key part of medical training and mentality. For example, soon after a patient presents to a doctor, their symptoms are quickly turned into a 'problem list' or differential diagnosis, which is likely to be tackled in a quantitative manner. Categorisation is accepted as common practice; it is therefore not surprising that these procedures are also used when it comes to individual patients, their ethnicities and their presumed religions. As Shaw states, a common response to difference in the consulting room is derived from standardised protocols. Although this can, at first glance, seem to be helpful in that it provides a clear mode of interaction with patients from different ethnic backgrounds, there is a highly paradoxical element to this: in essence, difference is dealt with by making things the same. Health professionals can expect to have standardised guidelines to inform them about the health or religious beliefs of a 'Muslim', an 'Asian' or 'African-Caribbean' patient or carer. Significantly, such a view undermines a neo-liberal shift within health policy in recent years that celebrates greater individual choice and the new rhetoric of 'no decision about me without me' (Department of Health 2006, 2009).

Chattoo points out that, although training in awareness of different social, cultural and religious backgrounds is important, recognition of each patient as an individual first and foremost is essential. She warns of the ease with which generalisations might be made based on ethnicity and the consequent loss of sensitivity regarding the particular socio-cultural world that each patient actually inhabits, rather than the one they are assumed to inhabit. Importantly, as Shaw shows in her chapter, it is very common for health care professionals to assume that culture and religion will directly inform and direct a South Asian patient's views of treatment, while the same assumptions are rarely applied to white patients. In that sense also, the 'culture' of Caucasian patients, as well as that of health care professionals, is rendered invisible, while that of patients of other ethnicities is often essentialised and problematised. Health care professionals therefore face the inherent dilemma of not passing judgement about individual patients based on ethnicity, while at the same time needing to be aware of the possible impact that culture and religion may have on views of treatment for patients of all ethnic backgrounds (including white British).

Practical Barriers: Language, Time and Policy Constraints

Negotiating cultural differences often comes hand in hand with practical issues of language competence, time and resource constraints. In practice, due to limitations in service provision, there may be difficulties in accessing interpreters, should they be required. In this case, a relative of the patient with greater command of English often takes the role of interpreter, thereby compromising patient confidentiality. This use of lay interpreters can cause further difficulties as the information may not be translated accurately, in both directions (Mir et al. 2001). In practice, translation is not only from one version of a language to another but also may entail further translation into a local dialect. For example, during clinical duties, one of us encountered a Chinese patient needing to be sectioned under the Mental Health Act due to severe depression. There were no translators who spoke his particular dialect. Because of this, the psychiatrist spoke in English to a translator, who translated into Cantonese for the patient's daughter, who then translated it into the local dialect for the patient. It was apparent that the greater the number of people required for the translation process, the more challenging it became to portray the meaning of the conversation, and maintain privacy. There were also difficulties with culturally bound ideas and terminology such as 'depression' and 'sadness' versus the abdominal pain that the patient complained of. This highlighted that communication between the health care professional and patient may also be impeded, not only by linguistic differences, but also by cultural differences in the way that the body and mind are understood and that sensitive issues are discussed. This is particularly relevant with ARTs, which both raises potentially very sensitive issues and also involves a complex interaction between perceptions of the body, kinship and societal expectations. These aspects of ARTs may not be easily translated between cultures or languages, and highlight the importance of facilitating these interactions in a sensitive manner and without presupposition.

Socio-cultural awareness and cultural competence must be implemented at both individual and policy levels, as there are implications both for individual health care decisions and for broader service provision. Although the training of health care professionals is key to the development of a more culturally competent workforce, these skills can only be put into practice within the wider constraints of the health care system. The complexity of the interaction is often compounded by time and resource constraints, which mean there may be little opportunity to explore a patient's concerns, let alone their socio-cultural background.

Despite having a particular interest in cultural diversity and health care, as a junior doctor it is often far too easy to neglect these issues as a result of the pressures of hospital life: staffing issues, time pressures, endless task lists and ever more seemingly urgent tasks to undertake. In order to allow culturally competent doctors to implement their skills, room must be made to do this. For example, increasing appointment lengths, especially when a sensitive or difficult topic might be anticipated, could allow the time to fully explore issues and personal beliefs and preferences, resulting in greater equity in treatment and outcome, and to render health care provision more culturally appropriate for all patients. This points to the need for flexibility within the health care system. It could be argued that investing in a more flexible system, although expensive in the short term, could bear long-term cost and policy benefits, as well as better treatment outcomes and greater patient satisfaction.

From Medical School to Practice as Junior Doctors: Medical Education and Training in Cultural Competence

In an earlier publication, Chattoo and Atkin (2012) highlighted the importance of linking the debates within social sciences with practical outcomes in improving culturally competent care in practice. Although there are still systemic policy issues that need to be addressed in terms of discrepancies in health and welfare provision, there have been significant improvements and changes in medical education over the last decade. Within increasingly globalised medical workforces and patient groups, which are also diverse in their constitution, there is an understanding that doctors need additional training to facilitate competence when dealing with diverse constituencies As Shaw argues, to implement cultural competence in practice, it is necessary to equip health care professionals with skills to work with diverse groups of patients. Below, we focus on our experiences of current medical education in the UK, providing a commentary on progress and ongoing difficulties in cultural competence training.

Cultural competency, as it is currently taught within medical education in the UK, covers three areas: cultural sensitivity, cultural knowledge and cultural skills. Although some integration of the first two has occurred, in our experience the teaching of cultural skills in medical education is still underdeveloped. However, there are opportunities to integrate, or offer opportunities for, cultural competence training. Within the core curriculum, some medical schools now have entire modules dedicated to social science approaches to social context and diversity, and their impact on a patient's health and well-being. As an example of the importance of teaching about culture in relation to illness in medical curricula, Newcastle Medical School uses in-depth patient studies to explore the impact of society and culture on health (and vice versa). Within the first year of training, each student follows a mother through her pregnancy and postpartum period, visiting her at her home on multiple occasions and thus getting a sense of how day-to-day life connects with the health care profession. This offers an unparalleled opportunity to explore the experiences and emotions of a woman and family who may have been through ART. Such training is essential to future practice, particularly when treating patients from widely different cultural backgrounds and practising in ethnically diverse neighbourhoods. However, these attempts at teaching about ethnic diversity can still result in 'us–them' dichotomies, particularly if theoretical knowledge is not appropriately balanced with practical implementation, in which case cultural awareness can become yet another 'factual' piece of information to remember rather than a skill set.

As mentioned earlier, a health care professional's own cultural constructs and background will affect patient interactions. This aspect of medical practice is rarely mentioned during medical education or training, and yet without understanding one's own beliefs and value structures and, indeed, recognising that allopathic medicine is an ethno-cultural product in itself, it is almost impossible to understand interaction with others from different backgrounds. One approach to remedying this issue might be a compulsory period of training either in a different country or in another social setting with which the student is unfamiliar. Indeed, in most medical schools during the senior years there is a medical elective period, during which students can spend a period of time practising medicine abroad. This can range from exposure to a 'state of the art' children's hospital in Canada, a clinic in the slums of Mumbai or a rural village in Malawi. Such electives can provide an opportunity to put theory into practice with exposure to different cultures and practices, settings, disease patterns and varied resource settings, thus providing an accelerated induction into the art of cultural competence. However, without a sound theoretical base in social sciences (for example sociology or anthropology), students can often struggle to make sense of the health disparities and cultural differences they encounter.

Many medical schools now also offer students the opportunity to intercalate – to take a year out of their course in order to pursue a further degree in a related subject. Traditionally this has often entailed the completion of a BSc or MSc in a scientific discipline such as biochemistry, physiology or microbiology but, in more recent years, there has been expansion into other subjects such as medical anthropology and global health. Such developments undoubtedly have the potential to increase those students' cultural awareness and cultural sensitivity. Encouragingly, there are an increasing number of students interested in global health (clinical and non-clinical aspects) and involved in activities outside the curriculum, with student groups such as 'Medsin' (Medical Students' International Network) in the UK, and the International Federation of Medical Students' Associations (IFMSA) worldwide, advocating, educating and acting upon global health issues. Within these larger umbrella groups there are also smaller projects aimed at specific areas within global health, such as 'Crossing Borders': an international network of students aiming to remove barriers to health care for refugees, asylum seekers and undocumented migrants. These initiatives, based in the UK, raise awareness of the importance of global health at home, and local initiatives that have a wider global impact. They also have the potential to equip students with skills to deal with cultural differences within local populations.

Following medical school, junior doctors attend weekly teaching sessions covering a wide range of subjects, and take part in professional days that occasionally touch upon subjects such as equality and diversity. However, these rarely attempt to unpick the intricacies of cultural competence within a health care context in any detail, and there is no current training focusing on cultural competence within these weekly teaching sessions. Therefore much more work still needs to be done to integrate and embed a culturally competent practice within health care professionals' everyday work, and to make more explicit the links between social and cultural diversity 'at home' and the increasingly globalised nature of health issues and health care practices more widely.

Conclusion

With an increasingly diverse population in the UK, it is vital that health care professionals are equipped to engage constructively, meaningfully and effectively with the cultural diversity of patients. In the process of training health care professionals to be culturally competent practitioners and enabling the implementation of these skills, flexibility needs to be a priority. In training future health care professionals, we argue that a more solid base in the social sciences is essential. Through these means we will be able to equip health care professionals with the appropriate skill sets and approaches to medical care that are cross-culturally transferable in ethnically diverse settings at home or abroad.

Ana Liddie Navarro is a junior doctor practising obstetrics and gynaecology in Northumberland, UK. She received her medical degree from Newcastle University in 2013, having obtained an MSc in Medical Anthropology from Durham University in 2012.

She has worked for the UK Medical Research Council researching mothers' access to health care for their children in The Gambia.

Miriam Orcutt (MBBS, MSc) is an academic foundation doctor in epidemiology and public health at the RVI, Newcastle upon Tyne, and a clinical research associate at the Institute of Health and Society, Newcastle University. A graduate from the MSc course in medical anthropology at Durham University, her fieldwork and dissertation focused on maternal mortality and access to health care in Eastern Zambia. Miriam has a keen interest in conflict and catastrophe medicine, emergency humanitarian response, and refugee and women's health. She aims to work in global public health and humanitarian aid.

Joint Bibliography

Abbasi-Shavazi, J., M. Inhorn, H.B. Razeghi-Nasrabad and G. Toloo. 2008. 'The "Iranian ART Revolution": Infertility, Assisted Reproductive Technology, and Third-Party Donation in the Islamic Republic of Iran', *Journal of Middle East Women's Studies* 4(2): 1–28.

Abbasi-Shavazi, J., H.B. Razeghi, Z.B. Ardekani and M.N. Akhondi. 2006. 'The Socio-cultural Aspects of Gamete and Embryo Donation in Infertility Treatment', in M.A. Akondi (ed), *Essays in Gamete and Embryo Donation in Infertility Treatment: From Medical, Theological, Legal, Ethical, Psychological and Sociological Approaches*. Tehran: Centre for Research and Development in Human Sciences (Semat), pp. 371–91.

Aboulghar, M.A. 2005. 'The Importance of Fertility Treatment in the Developing World', *British Journal of Obstetrics and Gynaecology* 112(9): 1174–76.

Adams, E. 2007. 'You Get On a Rollercoaster Where You Can't Get Off: Treatment Decision Making and "Choice" in the Context of Infertility after Breast Cancer', *Feminism and Psychology* 17(3): 330–35.

Ahmad, F. 2006. 'The Scandal of "Arranged Marriages" and the Pathologisation of BrAsian Families', in N. Ali, V.S. Kalra and S. Sayyid (eds), *A Postcolonial People: South Asians in Britain*. London: Hurst, pp. 272–88.

Ahmad, F., T. Modood and S. Lissenburgh. 2003. *South Asian Women and Employment in Britain: The Intersection of Gender and Ethnicity*. London: PSI.

Akondi, M.A. (ed.). 2001. *Modern Human Reproductive Techniques from the View of Jurisprudence and Law* (in Persian). The Avicenna Research Institute in association with the Academic Publishing House for the Social Sciences.

———. 2006. *Essays on Gamete and Embryo Donation in Infertility Treatment: From Medical, Theological, Legal, Ethical, Psychological and Sociological Approaches*. The Avicenna Research Institute in association with the Academic Publishing House for the Social Sciences.

American College of Obstetricians and Gynecologists. 2011. 'Effective Patient–Physician Communication'. Committee Opinion No. 492. *Obstet Gynecol* 117:1254–57.

Amin, N.S. 1996. *The World of Muslim Women in Colonial Bengal 1876–1939*. Leiden: Brill.

Anderson, B. 1991. *Imagined Communities: Reflections on the Origin and Spread of Nationalism*. London: Verso.

Anthias, F., and N. Yuval-Davis. 1992. *Racialised Boundaries: Race, Nation, Gender, Colour and Class and the Anti-Racist Struggle*. London and New York: Routledge.

Appadurai, A. 1996. *Modernity at Large: Cultural Dimensions of Globalization*. Minneapolis and London: University of Minnesota Press.

Arnfred, S. 2004. 'African Sexuality/Sexuality in Africa: Tales and Silences', in S. Arnfred (ed.), *Re-thinking Sexualities in Africa*. Uppsala: The Nordic Africa Institute, pp. 59–76.

Atighetchi, D. 2007. *Islamic Bioethics: Problems and Perspectives*. Dordrecht: Springer.

Atkin, K. 2004. 'Institutional Racism, Policy and Practice', in S. Ali and K. Atkin (eds), *Primary Healthcare and South Asian Populations: Meeting the Challenges*. Abingdon: Radcliffe, pp. 9–20.

Atkin, K., S. Ahmed, J. Green and J. Hewison. 2008. 'Decision-Making and Ante-Natal Screening for Sickle Cell and Thalassaemia Disorders: To What Extent Do Faith and Religious Identity Mediate Choice?', *Current Sociology* 56(1): 77–98.

Atkin, K., and E. Anionwu. 2010. 'The Social Consequences of Sickle Cell and Thalassaemia: Improving the Quality of Support', *Better Health Briefing Paper* 17. London: Race Equality Foundation, pp. 1–7.

Atkin, K., and S. Chattoo. 2007. 'The Dilemmas of Providing Welfare in an Ethnically Diverse State: Seeking Reconciliation in the Role of a "Reflexive Practitioner"', *Policy and Politics* 35(3): 379–95.

Baetens, P. et al. 2000. 'Counselling Couples and Donors for Oocyte Donation: The Decision to Use Either Known or Anonymous Oocytes', *Human Reproduction* 15(2): 476–84.

Bakhtin, M. 1981. *The Dialogic Imagination: Four Essays by Mikhail Bakhtin*, trans. C. Emerson and M. Holquist. Austin: University of Texas Press.

Baluch, B., A. Fallone and J. Khan. 1994. 'Gender Differences and Personality Correlates in Attitudes towards Controversial Aspects of Human Reproduction', *Journal of Social Behavior and Personality* 9(2): 329–34.

Bari, M.A. 2002. *Building Muslim Families: Challenges and Expectations*. London: Ta Ha Publishers Ltd.

Barkat, A., and M. Majid. 2003. *Adolescent and Youth Reproductive Health in Bangladesh: Status, Policies, Programs, and Issues*. Policy Project Report. Retrieved on 5 June 2014 from: www.policyproject.com/pubs/countryreports/ARH_Bangladesh.pdf

Barth, F. 2000. 'Boundaries and Connections', in A.P. Cohen (ed.), *Signifying Identities: Anthropological Perspectives on Boundaries and Contested Values*. London: Routledge, pp. 17–36.

Bauman, Z. 1992. *Intimations of Post Modernity*. London: Routledge.

Baumann, G. 1997. 'Dominant and Demotic Discourses of Culture: Their Relevance to Multi-Ethnic Alliances', in P. Werbner and T. Modood (eds), *Debating Cultural Hybridity: Multi-Cultural Identities and the Politics of Anti-Racism*. London: Zed Books, pp. 209–25.

BBC News. 2012. 'Funding IVF in the UK is Feeble'. Retrieved on 21 May 2013 from http://www.bbc.co.uk/news/health-18675858.

BBS (Bangladesh Bureau of Statistics). 2012. *Bangladesh 2011 Population & Housing Census: Final Result*, June. Retrieved 8 June 2014 from http://www.bbs.gov.bd/PageSecureReport.aspx

Beck, S. 2012. 'Biomedical Mobilities: Transnational Lab-Benches and Other Space Effects', in M. Knecht, M. Klotz and S. Beck (eds), *Reproductive Technologies as Global Form*. Chicago: Campus Press and University of Chicago Press, pp. 357–74.

Beck, U., and E. Beck-Gernsheim. 1995. *The Normal Chaos of Love*. Cambridge: Polity Press.

Becker, G. 2000. *The Elusive Embryo: How Women and Men Approach New Reproductive Technologies*. Berkeley: University of California Press.

Berer, M. 1999. 'Living Without Children', *Reproductive Health Matters* 7(13): 7–12.

Berthoud, R. 2005. 'Family Formation in Multi-cultural Britain: Diversity and Change', in G. Lowry, T. Modood and S. Teles, *Ethnicity, Social Mobility and Public Policy*. Cambridge: Cambridge University Press, pp. 222–52.

Beutel, M., J. Kupfer, P. Kirchmeyer and S. Kehde. 1998. 'Treatment-Related Stresses and Depression in Couples Undergoing Assisted Reproductive Treatment by IVF or ICSI', *Andrologia* 31(1): 27–36.

Beynon, H., D. Sadler and R. Hudson. 1994. *A Place Called Teesside: A Locality in a Global Economy*. Edinburgh: Edinburgh University Press,.

Bhabha, H. 1994. *The Location of Culture*. London: Routledge.

Bharadwaj, A. 2000 'How Some Indian Baby Makers Are Made: Media Narrative and Assisted Conception in India', *Anthropology and Medicine* 7(1): 70–78.

———. 2003.'Why Adoption is Not an Option in India: The Visibility of Infertility, the Secrecy of Donor Insemination, and Other Cultural Complexities', *Social Science & Medicine* 56(9): 1867–80.

———. 2008. 'Biosociality and Biocrossings: Encounters with Assisted Conception and Embryonic Stem Cells in India', in S. Gibbon and C. Novas (eds), *Biosocialities, Genetics and the Social Sciences: Making Biologies and Identities*. New York: Routledge, pp. 98–116.

Bhattacharji, S. 1983. *Ancient India: Society and Literature*, trans. Prachin Bharot: Somaj O shahitto. Calcutta: Anondo Publisher.

Bhatti, L.I., F.F. Fikree and A. Khan. 1999. 'The Quest of Infertile Women in Squatter Settlements of Karachi, Pakistan: A Qualitative Study', *Social Science & Medicine* 49(5): 637–49.

Bhui, K., N. Warfal, P. Edonyal, K. McKenzie, K. and D. Bhugra. 2007. 'Cultural Competence in Mental Health Care', *BMC Health Services Research* 7(15).

Bledsoe, C. 2002. *Contingent Lives: Fertility, Time and Aging in West Africa*. Chicago: University of Chicago Press.

Blerkom, J.V., et al. 2014 'First Births with a Simplified Culture System for Clinical IVF and Embryo Transfer', *Reproductive BioMedicine Online* 28(3): 310–20.

Blyth, E., L. Frith and A. Farrand. 2005. 'Is It Possible to Recruit Gamete Donors Who Are Both Altruistic and Identifiable?', *Fertility and Sterility* 84(S1): S21–S22.

Blyth, E., and R. Landau (eds). 2004. *Third Party Assisted Conception across Cultures: Social, Legal and Ethical Perpectives*. London: Routledge.

Böck, M., and A. Rao. 2000. *Culture, Creation and Procreation: Concepts of Kinship in South Asian Practice*. Oxford and New York: Berghahn Books.

Boivin, J., L. Bunting, J.A. Collins and K.G. Nygren. 2007. 'International Estimates of Infertility Prevalence and Treatment-Seeking: Potential Need and Demand for Infertility Medical Care', *Human Reproduction* 22(6): 1506–12.

Boivin, J., and L. Schmidt. 2005. 'Infertility-Related Stress in Men and Women Predicts Treatment Outcome One Year Later', *Fertility and Sterility* 83(6): 1745–52.

Bolton, V., S. Golombok, R. Cook and J. Rust. 1991. 'A Comparative Study of Attitudes towards Donor Insemination and Egg Donation in Recipients, Potential Donors and the Public', *Journal of Psychosomatic Obstetrics and Gynecology* 12: 217–28.

Bonaccorso-Rothe, M.E. 2009. *Conceiving Kinship: Assisted Conception, Procreation and Family in Southern Europe*. Oxford: Berghahn Books.

Bradby, H. 2003. 'Describing Ethnicity in Health Research', *Ethnicity and Health* 8(1): 5–13.

Brah, A. 1996. *Cartographies of Diaspora: Contesting Identities*. London: Routledge.

Brett, S., R. Sacranie, G. Thomas and R. Rajkhowa. 2008. 'Can We Improve Recruitment of Oocyte Donors with Loss of Donor Anonymity? A Hospital Based Survey', *Human Fertility* 11: 101–7.

Brockopp, J. (ed.). 2003. *Islamic Ethics of Life: Abortion, War, and Euthanasia*. Columbia: University of South Carolina Press.

Brockopp, J., and T. Eich (eds). 2008. *Muslim Medical Ethics: From Theory to Practice*. Columbia: University of South Carolina Press.

Browne, A. 2000. 'Whites Will be an Ethnic Minority in Britain by the End of the Century', *The Observer on Sunday*, 3 September.

Carmeli, Y.S., and D. Birenbaum-Carmeli. 2000. 'Ritualising the "Natural Family": Secrecy in Israeli Donor Insemination', *Science and Culture* 9: 301–24.

Carrithers, M. 2005. 'Why Anthropologists Should Study Rhetoric', *Journal of the Royal Anthropological Institute* 11(3): 577–83.

Carsten, J. (ed.). 2000. *Cultures of Relatedness: New Approaches to the Study of Kinship*. Cambridge: Cambridge University Press.

Cates, W., T.M. Farley and P.J. Rowe. 1985.'Worldwide Patterns of Infertility: Is Africa Different?' *Lancet* 2(8455): 596–98.

Chakravarty, B.N., and S.G. Dastidar. 1986. 'Our Experience of In Vitro Fertilisation and Embryo Transfer', *Journal of Obstetrics and Gynaecology of India* 36: 566–72.

Chapple, A., M. Salinas, S. Ziebland, A. McPherson and A. Macfarlane. 2007. 'Fertility Issues: The Perceptions and Experiences of Young Men Recently Diagnosed and Treated for Cancer', *Journal of Adolescent Health* 40(1): 69–75.

Charsley, K. 2005. 'Unhappy Husbands: Masculinity and Migration in Transnational Pakistani Marriages', *The Journal of the Royal Anthropological Institute* 11(1): 85–105.

Chattoo, S. 1990. *A Sociological Study of Certain Aspects of Disease and Death: A Case Study of Muslims of Kashmir*. PhD dissertation. Delhi: University of Delhi.

Chattoo, S., and W. Ahmad. 2008. 'The Moral Economy of Selfhood and Caring: Negotiating Boundaries of Personal Care as Embodied Moral Practice', *Sociology of Health and Illness* 30(4): 550–64.

Chattoo, S., W. Ahmad, M. Haworth and R. Lennard. 2002. 'South Asian and White Patients with Advanced Cancer: Patients' and Families' Experiences of the Illness and Perceived Needs for Care'. Final Report submitted to the Cancer Research UK and the Department of Health, Centre for Research in Primary Care, University of Leeds.

Chattoo, S., and K. Atkin. 2009. 'Extending Specialist Palliative Care to People with Heart Failure: Semantic, Historical and Practical Limitations to Policy Guidelines', *Social Science & Medicine* 69(2): 147–53.

———. 2012. 'Race, Ethnicity and Social Policy: Theoretical Concepts and Limitations of Current Approaches to Welfare', in G. Craig, K. Atkin, S. Chattoo and R. Flynn (eds), *Understanding 'Race' and Ethnicity in Social Welfare*. Bristol: Policy Press, pp. 19–40.

Chattoo, S., M. Crawshaw and K. Atkin. 2010. *The Experiences of Cancer-Related Fertility Impairment among People of South Asian and White Origin*. York: University of York.

Chinnatamby, S. 1970. 'Infertility Services in a Family Planning Clinic', *International Planned Parenthood Federation Medical Bulletin* 4: 3–4.

———. 1990. 'Role of Planned Parenthood for Enrichment of the Quality of Life in Sri Lanka', *Ceylon Medical Journal* 35: 136–42.

Chliaoutakis, J., Koukouli, S. and M. Papadakaki. 2002. 'Using Attitudinal Indicators to Explain the Public's Intention to Have Recourse to Gamete Donation and Surrogacy', *Human Reproduction* 17(11): 2995–3002.

Clarke, M. 2006. 'Islam, Kinship and New Reproductive Technology', *Anthropology Today* 22: 17–22.

———. 2007. 'Children of The Revolution: Ayatollah Khamene'i's "Liberal" Views on In Vitro Fertilisation', *British Journal of Middle Eastern Studies* 34(3): 287–303.

———. 2009. *Islam and New Kinship: Reproductive Technologies and the Shariah in Lebanon*. New York and Oxford: Berghahn Books.

———. 2010. 'Neo-Calligraphy: Religious Authority and Media Technology in Contemporary Shiite Islam', *Comparative Studies in Society and History* 52(2): 351–83.

———. 2012a. 'Islamic Bioethics and Religious Politics in Lebanon', in M. Inhorn and S. Tremayne (eds), *Islam and Assisted Reproductive Technologies: Sunni and Shia Perspectives*. New York: Berghahn Books, pp. 261–84.

———. 2012b. 'The Judge as Tragic Hero: Judicial Ethics in Lebanon's Sharia Courts', *American Ethnologist* 39(1): 101–16.

Clarke, M., and M.C. Inhorn. 2011. 'Mutuality and Immediacy between Marja' and Muqallid: Evidence from Male IVF Patients in Shi'i Lebanon', *International Journal of Middle East Studies* 43(3): 409–27.

Coleman, D., and S. Dubuc. 2010. 'The Fertility of Ethnic Minorities in the UK, 1960s–2006', *Population Studies* 64(1): 19–41.

Colen, S. 1986. '"With Respect and Feeling": Voices of West Indian Childcare and Domestic Workers in New York City', in J.B. Cole (ed.), *All American Women: Lives that Divide and Ties that Bind*. New York: Free Press, pp. 46–63.

———. 1995. '"Like a Mother to Them": Stratified Reproduction and West Indian Childcare Workers and Employers in New York', in Faye D. Ginsburg and Rayna Rapp (eds), *Conceiving the New World Order: The Global Politics of Reproduction*, pp. 78–102.

Culley, L., and N. Hudson. 2007. 'Public Understandings of Science: British South Asian Men's Perceptions of Third-Party Assisted Conception', *The International Journal of Interdisciplinary Social Sciences* 2(4): 79–86.

———. 2009a. 'Constructing Relatedness: Ethnicity, Gender and Third-Party Assisted Conception in the UK', *Current Sociology* 57(2): 257–75.

———. 2009b. 'Commonalities, Differences and Possibilities: Culture and Infertility in British South Asian Communities', in L. Culley, N. Hudson and F. van Rooij (eds), *Marginalized Reproduction: Ethnicity, Infertility and New Reproductive Technologies*. London: Earthscan, pp. 97–116.

Culley, L., N. Hudson and F. Rapport. 2007. 'Using Focus Groups with Minority Ethnic Communities: Researching Infertility in British South Asian Communities', *Qualitative Health Research* 17(1): 102–12.

Culley, L., N. Hudson, R. Rapport, E. Blyth, W. Norton and A.A. Pacey. 2011. 'Crossing Borders for Fertility Treatment: Motivations, Destinations and Outcomes of UK Fertility Travellers', *Human Reproduction* 26(9): 2373–81.

Culley, L., N. Hudson, F. Rapport, M. Johnson and A. Bharadwaj. 2006a. 'Public Perceptions of Gamete Donation in British South Asian Communities'. Report on ESRC Study. Leicester: De Montfort University.

Culley, L., N. Hudson, F. Rapport, S. Katbamna and M. Johnson. 2006b. 'British South Asian Communities and Infertility Services', *Human Fertility* 9(1): 37–45.

Culley, L., F. Rapport, S. Katbamna, M. Johnson and N. Hudson. 2004. 'A Study of the Provision of Infertility Services to South Asian Communities'. Final Report to NHS Executive Trent. Leicester: De Montfort University.

Cunningham-Burley, S., A. Kerr and S. Pavis. 2001. 'Focus Groups and Public Involvement in the New Genetics'. PLA notes (40). London: IIED.

Cussins, C.M. 1996. 'Ontological Choreography: Agency for Women Patients in an Infertility Clinic', in M. Berg and A. Mol (eds), *Differences in Medicine: Unravelling Practices, Techniques and Bodies*. Durham, NC: Duke University Press, pp. 166–201.

Daar, A.S., and Z. Merali. 2002. 'Infertility and Social Suffering: The Case of ART in Developing Countries', in E. Vayena, J.P. Rowe and P.D. Griffin (eds), *Current Practices and Controversies in Assisted Reproduction*. Geneva: World Health Organization, pp. 15–21.

Das, V. 1995. *Critical Events: An Anthropological Perspective on Contemporary India*. Oxford: Oxford University Press.

Das, V., and D. Poole. 2004. 'State and It's Margins: Comparative Ethnographies', in V. Das and D. Poole (eds), *Anthropology in the Margins of the State*. Oxford, New York and New Delhi: Oxford University Press, pp. 3–34.

Deeb, L. 2006. *An Enchanted Modern: Gender and Public Piety in Shi'i Lebanon*. Princeton, NJ: Princeton University Press.

Delius, P., and C. Glaser. 2005. 'Sex, Disease and Stigma in South Africa: Historical Perspectives', *African Journal of AIDS Research* 4(1): 29–36.

Department of Census and Statistics (DCS) and Ministry of Health Care and Nutrition. 2000. 'Demographic and Health Survey 2000'. Colombo, Sri Lanka.

———. 2009. 'Demographic and Health Survey 2006–7'. Colombo, Sri Lanka.

Department of Health. 2004. 'Anonymity to be Removed from Future Sperm, Egg and Embryo Donors'. Retrieved on 28 July from: http://www.dh.gov.uk/PublicationsAndStatistics/PressReleases/PressReleasesNotices/fs/en?CONTENT_ID=4070524&chk=jLTlI%2B

———. 2006. 'Choice Matters: Increasing Choice Improves People's Experiences'. London.

———. 2009. 'Your Health, Your Way: A Guide to Long-Term Conditions'. London.

———. 2010. Human Fertilisation and Embryology Act 2008 (Commencement) Order 2010. London.

———. 2012. Government Response to Consultation "Liberating the NHS: No decision about me, without me". London.

De Sutter, P. 2011. 'Considerations for Clinics and Practitioners Treating Foreign Patients with Assisted Reproductive Technology: Lessons from Experiences at Ghent University Hospital, Belgium', *Reproductive Biomedicine Online* 23: 652–56.

Dhont, N. 2011a. 'Clinical, Epidemiological and Socio-cultural Aspects of Infertility in Resource-Poor Settings', *Facts, Views and Visions in Ob/Gyn* 3(2): 77–88.

———. 2011b. 'The Walking Egg Non-Profit Organization', *Facts, Views & Vision in Ob/Gyn* 3(4): 253–55.

Dill, S.K. 2007. 'International Treatment Differences: Policy, Politics, Partnership and ART', *Pharmaceuticals Policy and Law* 9: 147–56.

Dissanayake, V.H.W., B. Simpson and R.W. Jayasekara. 2002. 'Attitudes towards the New Genetic and Assisted Reproductive Technologies in Sri Lanka: A Preliminary Report', *New Genetics and Society* 21(1): 65–74.

Donovan, C. 2006. 'Genetics, Fathers and Families: Exploring the Implications of Changing the Law in Favour of Identifying Sperm Donors', *Social & Legal Studies* 15(4): 494–510.

Draper, H., and J. Ives. 2009. 'Paternity Testing: A Poor Test of Fatherhood', *Journal of Social Welfare and Family Law* 31(4): 407–18.

Dyer, S.J., N. Abrahams, N.E. Mokoena and Z.M. van der Spuy. 2004.'"You Are a Man Because You Have Children": Experiences, Reproductive Health Knowledge and Treatment-Seeking Behaviour among Men Suffering from Couple Infertility in South Africa', *Human Reproduction* 19(4): 960–67.

Dyer, S., C. Lombard and Z. van der Spuy. 2009. 'Psychological Distress among Men Suffering from Couple Infertility in South Africa: A Quantitative Assessment', *Human Reproduction* 24(11): 2821–26.

Edouard, L., and O.A. Olatunbosun. 1997. 'Correspondence', *British Journal of Obstetrics and Gynaecology* 104(8): 969–74.

Edwards, J. 1993. 'Explicit Connections: Ethnographic Enquiry in North-West England', in J. Edwards, S. Franklin, E. Hirsch, F. Price and M. Strathern (eds), *Technologies of Procreation: Kinship in the Age of Assisted Conception*. London: Routledge, pp. 60–85.

———. 2002. 'Taking Public Understanding Seriously', *New Genetics and Society* 21(3): 315–25.

———. 2004. 'Incorporating Incest: Gamete, Body and Relation in Assisted Conception', *The Journal of the Royal Anthropological Institute* 10(4): 755–74.

———. 2009. 'Skipping a Generation and Assisting Conception', in S. Bamford and J. Leach (eds), *Kinship and Beyond: The Genealogical Model Reconsidered*. New York and Oxford: Berghahn Books, pp. 138–75.

Eich, T. 2012. 'Constructing Kinship in Sunni Islamic Legal Texts', in M. Inhorn and S. Tremayne (eds), *Islam and Assisted Reproductive Technologies: Sunni and Shia Perspectives*. New York and Oxford: Berghahn Books, pp. 27–52.

Ericksen, K., and T. Brunette. 1996. 'Patterns and Predictors of Infertility among African Women: A Cross-National Survey of Twenty-Seven Nations', *Social Science & Medicine* 42(2): 209–20.

ESHRE. 2012. 'The World's Number of IVF Babies has now Reached a Calculated Total of 5 Million', ESRHE Press Release. Retrieved 31 May 2014 from http//www.eshre.eu/press-room/press-releases/:ESRHE-2012/5-million-babies.aspx.

Farouk, M. 2010. 'Assisted Reproductive Technology (ART) – Ethics, Religion and the Law', *Sri Lanka Journal of Obstetrics and Gynaecology* 32: 49–52.

Fathalla, M.F., S.W. Sinding, A. Rosenfield and M.M. Fathalla. 2006. 'Sexual and Reproductive Health for All: A Call for Action', *Lancet* 368(9552): 2095–100.

Feldman-Savelsberg, P. 1999. *Plundered Kitchens, Empty Wombs: Threatened Reproduction and Identiy in the Cameroon Grassfields*. Ann Arbor: The University of Michigan Press.

Fenton, S. 2003. *Ethnicity*. Cambridge: Polity Press.

Ferraretti, A.P., et al. 2012. 'The European IVF-monitoring [EIM] and Consortium for the European Societey of Human Reproduction and Embryology (ESHRE). Assisted Reproductive Technology in Europe, 2008'. Retrieved 10 July 2012 from doi:10.1093/humrep/des255.

FIGO. 2003. 'Resolution on Professional and Ethical Responsibilities Concerning Sexual and Reproductive Rights', International Federation of Gynaecology and Obstetrics (FIGO). Retrieved 13 December 2012 from www.figo.org/projects/ethical_responsibility

Forrest, L., and L.G. Gilbert. 1992. 'Infertility: An Unanticipated and Prolonged Life Crisis', *Journal of Mental Health Counselling* 14: 42–58.

Franklin, S. 1995. 'Postmodern Procreation: A Cultural Account of Assisted Reproduction', in F.D. Ginsburg and R. Rapp (eds), *Conceiving the New World Order: The Global Politics of Reproduction*. Berkeley: University of California Press, pp. 323–45.

———. 1997. *Embodied Progress: A Cultural Account of Assisted Conception*. London: Routledge.

———. 2012. 'Five Million Miracle Babies Later: The Biocultural Legacies of IVF', in M. Knecht, M. Klotz and S. Beck (eds), *Reproductive Technologies as Global Form*. Chicago: Campus Press and University of Chicago Press, pp. 27–42.

Gaily, Z.M., E. Elhussein and Z. Karar. 2010. 'Short-Term Outcome of In-Vitro Fertilization Babies (IVF) in Sudan', *Sudanese Journal of Paediatrics and Child Health* 10: 28–31.

Gaonkar, D. (ed.). 2001. *Alternative Modernities*. Durham, NC: Duke University Press.

Garmaroudi, S. 2012. 'Gestational Surrogacy in Iran: Uterine Kinship in Shia Thought and Practice', in M. Inhorn and S. Tremayne (eds), *Islam and Assisted Reproductive Technologies: Sunni and Shia Perspectives*. New York: Berghahn Books, pp. 157–93.

Geertz, C. 1983. *Local Knowledge: Further Essays in Interpretative Anthropology*. New York: Basic Books.

Geest, S. van der, and P. Nahar. 2013. 'Understanding Life through Unwanted Childlessness: Ethnography and Fiction from Ghana, Bangladesh and "Dystopia"', *Anthropology Today* 29(3): 3–7.

Geissler, W., and R. Prince. 2007. 'Life Seen: Touch and Vision in the Making of Sex in Western Kenya', *Journal of Eastern African Studies* 1(1): 123–49.

Gelvin, James L. 2005. *The Modern Middle East: A History*. New York: Oxford University Press.

Gerrits, T. 1997. 'Social and Cultural Aspects of Infertility in Mozambique', *Patient Education and Counseling* 31(1): 39–48.

———. 2002. 'Infertility and Matrilineality: The Exceptional Case of the Macua of Mozambique', in M.C. Inhorn and F. Van Balen (eds), *Infertility around the Globe: New Thinking on Childlessness, Gender, and Reproductive Technologies*. Berkeley: University of California Press, pp. 233–46.

———. 2014. 'The Ambiguity of Patient-Centered Practices: The Case of a Dutch Fertility Clinic', *Anthropology and Medicine*. DOI: 10.1080/13648470.2014.914804.

Gerrits, T., and V. Hörbst (forthcoming). 'A Mercedes-Benz and a Chop Bar: Assisted Reproductive Technologies and Entrepreneurship in Ghana', in Lenore Manderson, Anita Hardon and Elizabeth Cartwright (eds), *Handbook of Medical Anthropology of the 21st Century*. London: Routledge.

Gerrits, T., and M. Shaw. 2010. 'Biomedical Infertility Care in Sub-Saharan Africa: A Social Science Review of Current Practices, Experiences and View Points', *Facts, Views & Visions in ObGyn* 2(3): 194–207.

Giddens, A. 1991. *Modernity and Self-Identity: Self and Society in the Late Modern Age*. Oxford: Polity Press.

Ginsburg, F.D., and R. Rapp. 1991. 'The Politics of Reproduction', *Annual Review of Anthropology* 20: 311–43.

———. 1995. 'Introduction: Conceiving the New World Order', in F. Ginsburg and R. Rapp (eds), *Conceiving the New World Order: The Global Politics of Reproduction*. Berkeley: University of California Press, pp. 1–17.

Glausiusz, J. 2009. 'Low-Cost IVF Comes to Africa', *New Scientist* 203(2723): 8–9.

Goldstein, J.R., T. Sobotka and A. Jasilioniene. 2009. 'The End of the "Lowest-Low" Fertility?', *Population and Demographic Review* 35(4): 663–99.

Golombok, S., and C. Murray. 1999. 'Egg and Semen Donation: A Survey of UK Licensed Centres'. Report for the National Gamete Donation Trust. London: City University.

Greil, A.L. 1991. *Not Yet Pregnant: Infertile Couple's Contemporary America*. New Brunswick, NJ: Rutgers University Press.

Greil, A.L., K. Slauson-Blevins and J. McQuillan. 2010. 'The Experience of Infertility: A Review of Recent Literature', *Sociology of Health and Illness* 32(1): 140–62.

Gunaratnam, Y. 2008. 'From Competence of Vulnerability: Care, Ethics and Elders from Racialized Minorities', *Mortality* 13(1): 24–41.

Guntupalli, A.M., and P. Chenchelgudem. 2004. 'Perceptions, Causes and Consequences of Infertility among the Chanchu Tribe of India', *Journal of Reproductive and Infant Psychology* 22(4): 249–59.

Gupta, J.A. 2000. *New Reproductive Technologies, Women's Health and Autonomy: Freedom or Dependency?* New Delhi: Sage.

———. 2005. 'Local Articulation of Globalized Assisted Reproduction Technologies in the Socio-Cultural Context of India', in R.N. Pakti and N.K. Pati (eds), *Population Challenges and Health: Needs in Orissa*. Orissa: The Home of Letters, pp. 155–71.

———. 2006. 'Towards Transnational Feminism: Some Reflections and Concerns in Relation to the Globalization of Reproductive Technologies', *European Journal of Women's Studies* 13(1): 23–38.

Gupta, J.A., and A. Richters. 2008. 'Embodied Subjects and Fragmented Objects: Women's Bodies, Assisted Reproduction Technologies and the Right to Self-Determination', *Bioethical Inquiry* 5: 239–49.

Haimes, E. 1993. 'Issues of Gender in Gamete Donation', *Social Science & Medicine* 36(1): 85–93.

Hall, S. 1996. 'Introduction: Who Needs Identity', in S. Hall and P. du Gay (eds), *Questions of Cultural Identity*. London: Sage, pp. 1–7.

Hallaq, W. 2009. *Shari'a: Theory, Practice, Transformations*. Cambridge: Cambridge University Press.

Hamberger, L., and P.O. Janson. 1997. 'Global Importance of Infertility and its Treatment: Role of Fertility Technologies', *International Journal of Gynaecology and Obstetrics* 58(1): 149–58.

Hamilton, M. 2010. 'Sperm Donation in the United Kingdom in 2010', *Human Fertility* 13(4): 257–62.

Hampshire, K., M. Blell and B. Simpson. 2012a. '"Everybody is Moving On": Infertility, Relationality and the Aesthetics of Family among British-Pakistani Muslims', *Social Science & Medicine* 74(7): 1045–52.

———. 2012b. 'Navigating New Socio-Demographic Landscapes: Using Anthropological Demography to Explain the "Persistence" of High and Early Fertility among British Pakistanis', *European Journal of Population / Revue européenne de Démographie* 28(1): 39.

Hampshire, K., N. Iqbal, M. Blell and B. Simpson. 2014. The Interview as Narrative Ethnography: Seeking and Shaping Connections in Qualitative Research', *International Journal of Social Research Methodology* 17(3): 215–31.

Handwerker L. 2002. 'The Politics of Making Modern Babies in China: Reproductive Technologies and the "New" Eugenics', in M.C. Inhorn and F. Van Balen (eds), *Infertility around the Globe: New Thinking on Childlessness, Gender, and Reproductive Technologies*. Berkeley: University of California Press, pp. 298–314.

Haq, E.M. 1976. *History of Sufism in Bengal*. Dhaka: The Asiatic Society of Bangladesh.

Harcourt, W. 1997. 'Introduction', in W. Harcourt (ed.), *Power, Reproduction and Gender: The Intergenerational Transfer of Knowledge*. London: Zed Books, pp. 1–7.

Harik, J. 2006. 'Hizballah's Public and Social Services and Iran', in H. Chehabi (ed.), *Distant Relations: Iran and Lebanon in the Last 500 Years*. London: Centre for Lebanese Studies in association with I.B. Tauris, pp. 259–86.

Harriss, K., and A. Shaw. 2009. 'Kinship Obligations, Gender and the Life Course: Re-Writing Migration from Pakistan to Britain', V. Kalra (ed.), *Pakistani Diasporas: Culture, Conflict and Change*. Oxford: Oxford University Press, pp. 105–28.

Hess, D. 1994. 'Parallel Universes: Anthropology in the World of Technoscience', *Anthropology Today* 10: 16–18.

Hesse, B., and B. Sayyid. 2006. 'Narrating the Postcolonial Political and the Immigrant Imaginary', in N. Ali, V.S. Kalra and S. Sayyid (eds), *A Postcolonial People: South Asians in Britain*. London: Hurst, pp. 13–31.

Human Fertilisation and Embryology Authority (HFEA). 2006. 'SEED Report: A Report on the Human Fertilisation & Embryology Authority's Review of Sperm, Egg and Embryo Donation in the United Kingdom'. London.

———. 2007. 'Human Fertilisation and Embryology Annual IVF Figures for 2006'. Retrieved on 12 July 2012 from http://www.hfea.gov.uk/ivf-figures-2006.html#1278

———. 2011a. 'Fertility Treatment in 2010: Trends and Figures'. Retrieved on 12 January 2012 from http://www.hfea.gov.uk/6771.html

———. 2011b. 'HFEA Agrees New Policies to Improve Sperm and Egg Services'. Retrieved on 12 January 2012 from: http//www.hfea.gov.uk/6700.html

Hirsch, E. 1999. 'Negotiated Limits: Interviews in South-East England', in J. Edwards, S. Franklin, E. Hirsch, F. Price and M. Strathern (eds), *Technologies of Procreation: Kinship in the Age of Assisted Conception*, 2nd edn. Manchester: Manchester University Press, pp. 91–121.

Holquist, M. 2002. *Dialogism: Bakhtin and His World*, 2nd edn. London and New York: Routledge.

Holter, H., L. Anderheim, C. Bergh and A. Moller. 2006. 'First IVF Treatment: Short-Term Impact on Psychological Well-Being and the Marital Relationship', *Human Reproduction* 21(12): 3295–302.

Hörbst, V. 2006. 'Infertility and In-vitro Fertilization in Bamako, Mali: Women's Experience, Avenues for Solution and Social Contexts Impacting on Gynaecological Consultations', *Curare* 29(1): 35–46.

———. 2010. 'Male Perspectives on Infertility and Assisted Reproductive Technologies (ART) in sub-Saharan Contexts', *Facts, Views & Visions in ObGyn* 2(3): 22–27.

———. 2012. 'Assisted Reproductive Technologies in Mali: Asymmetries and Frictions', in M. Knecht, M. Klotz and S. Beck (eds), *IVF as Global*

Form: Ethnographies of Knowledge, Practices, and Transnational Encounters. New York: Campus, pp. 120–48.

Hörbst, V., and T. Gerrits (forthcoming). 'Transnational Connections of Health Professionals: Mobility, Networks, and Assisted Reproduction in Sub-Saharan Africa (in Ghana and Uganda)', *Ethnicity and Health*.

Hörbst, V., and A. Wolf. 2014. 'ARVs and ARTs: Medicoscapes and the Unequal Place-making for Biomedical Treatments in Sub-Saharan Africa', *Medical Anthropology Quarterly* 28(2): 182–202.

Horst, H., and D. Miller. 2006. *The Cell Phone: An Anthropology of Communication*. Oxford: Berg.

Hudson, N. 2008. 'Infertility in British South Asian Communities: Negotiating the Community and the Clinic', PhD dissertation. Leicester: De Montfort University.

Hudson, N., L. Culley, F. Rapport, M. Johnson and A. Bharadwaj. 2009. '"Public" Perceptions of Gamete Donation: A Research Review', *Public Understanding of Science* 18(1): 61–77.

Hull, M.G.R., C.M.A. Galzener and N.J. Kelly. 1985, 'Population Study of Causes, Treatment and Outcome of Infertility', *British Medical Journal* 291(54): 1693–97.

Hunt, N.R. 2005. 'Fertility Fires and Empty Wombs in Recent Africanist Writing', *Africa* 75(3): 421–35.

ICPD. 1994. 'Report of the International Conference on Population and Development'. United Nations Population Information Network. Retrieved 30 May 2014 from http://www.un.org/popin/icpd/conference/offeng/poa.html.

Ingerslev, H.J., A. Hojgaard, J. Hindkjaer and U. Kesmodel. 2001. 'A Randomized Study Comparing IVF in the Unstimulated Cycle with IVF Following Clomiphene Citrate', *Human Reproduction* 16(4): 696–702.

Inhorn, M.C. 1994a. *Quest for Conception: Gender, Infertility and Egyptian Medical Traditions*. Philadelphia: University of Pennsylvania Press.

———. 1994b. 'Interpreting Infertility: Medical Anthropology Perspectives', *Social Science & Medicine* 39(4): 459–61.

———. 1996. *Infertility and Patriarchy: The Cultural Politics of Gender and Family Life in Egypt*. Philadelphia: University of Pennsylvania Press.

———. 2002. 'The "Local" Confronts the "Global": Infertile Bodies and New Reproductive Technologies in Egypt', in M.C. Inhorn and F. Van Balen (eds), *Infertility around the Globe: New Thinking on Childlessness, Gender, and Reproductive Technologies*. Berkeley: University of California Press, pp. 263–82.

———. 2003a. 'The Worms Are Weak – Male Infertility and Patriarchal Paradoxes in Egypt', *Men and Masculinities* 5(3): 236–56.

———. 2003b. *Local Babies, Global Science: Gender, Religion, and In Vitro Fertilization in Egypt*. New York: Routledge.

———. 2003c. 'Global Infertility and the Globalization of New Reproductive Technologies: Illustrations from Egypt', *Social Science & Medicine* 56(9): 1837–51.

———. 2004. 'Middle Eastern Masculinities in the Age of New Reproductive Technologies: Male Infertility and Stigma in Egypt and Lebanon', *Medical Anthropology Quarterly* 18(2): 34–54.

———. 2005. 'Fatwas and ARTS: IVF and Gamete Donation in Sunni v. Shi'a Islam', *Journal of Gender, Race and Justice* 9(2): 291–318.

———. 2006a. "He Won't Be My Son': Middle Eastern Muslim Men's Discourses of Adoption and Gamete Donation', *Medical Anthropology Quarterly* 20(1): 94–120.

———. 2006b. 'Making Muslim Babies: IVF and Gamete Donation in Sunni versus
Shi'a Islam', *Culture, Medicine and Psychiatry* 30: 427–50.

———. 2007a. 'Masturbation, Semen Collection and Men's IVF Experiences: Anxieties in the Muslim World', *Body and Society* 13(3): 37–53.

——— (ed.). 2007b. *Reproductive Disruptions: Gender, Technology and Biopolitics in the New Millennium*. New York: Berghahn Books.

———. 2009. 'Right to Assisted Reproductive Technology: Overcoming Infertility in Low-Resource Countries', *International Journal of Gynecology and Obstetrics* 106: 172–74.

———. 2011. 'Globalization and Gametes: Reproductive 'Tourism', Islamic Bioethics, and Middle Eastern Modernity', *Anthropology and Medicine* 18(1): 87–103.

———. 2012. *The New Arab Man: Emergent Masculinities, Technologies, and Islam in the Middle East*. Princeton, NJ: Princeton University Press.

Inhorn, M.C., and D. Birenbaum-Carmeli. 2008. 'Assisted Reproductive Technologies and Culture Change', *Annual Review of Anthropology* 37: 177–96.

Inhorn, M.C., and Z.B. Gürtin. 2011. Cross-Border Reproductive Care: A Future Research Agenda, *Reproductive Biomedicine Online* 23(5): 665–76.

Inhorn, M.C., and P. Patrizio. 2009. 'Rethinking Reproductive "Tourism" as Reproductive "Exile"', *Fertility and Sterility* 92(3): 904–6.

Inhorn, M.C., P. Patrizio and G. Serour. 2010. 'Third-Party Reproductive Assistance around the Mediterranean: Comparing Sunni Egypt, Catholic Italy and Multi-Sectarian Lebanon', *Reproductive Medicine Online* 21(7): 848–53.

Inhorn, M.C., and S. Tremayne (eds). 2012. *Islam and Assisted Reproductive Technologies: Sunni and Shia Perspectives*. New York and Oxford: Berghahn Books.

Inhorn M.C., and F. Van Balen (eds). 2002. *Infertility around the Globe: New Thinking on Childlessness, Gender and Reproductive Technologies*. Berkeley: University of California Press.

Iqbal, N. 2009. 'Fluidity, Subjectivity and Choice: The Practice of Relatedness among British Pakistani Muslims'. PhD disssertation. Durham: University of Durham.

Isikoglu, M., Y. Senol, M. Berkkanoglu, K. Ozgur, L. Donmez and A. Stones-Abbasi. 2006. 'Public Opinion Regarding Oocyte Donation in

Turkey: First Data from a Secular Population among the Islamic World', *Human Reproduction* 21(1): 318–23.

IVF.net. 2014. 'IVF Net – IVF Clinics'. Retrieved on 1 May 2014 from http://www.ivf.net/ivf/clinics-b360.html

Jacobson-Widding, A., and W. Van Beek. 1990. *The Creative Communion: African Folk Models of Fertility and the Regeneration of Life*. Uppsala: Almqvist and Wiksell.

Johnson, M.H., J. Cohen and G. Grudszinskas. 2014 'Accessible and Affordable IVF: Is Bob Edwards' Dream about to Become Reality?', *Reproductive Biomedicine Online* 28(3): 265–66.

Johnson-Hanks, J. 2002. 'On the Modernity of Traditional Contraception: Time and the Social Context of Fertility', *Population and Development Reviews* 28(2): 229–48

Jonsen, A. 1998. *The Birth of Bioethics*. New York: Oxford University Press.

Kahn, S.M. 2000. *Reproducing Jews: A Cultural Account of Assisted Conception in Israel*. Durham, NC: Duke University Press.

Kailasam, C., K. Sykes and J. Jenkins. 2001. 'A Survey of Public Attitudes to Gamete Donation', *Journal of Fertility Counselling* 8(2): 45–48.

Kan, A.K., H.I. Abdalla, B.O. Ogunyemi, L. Korea and E. Latarche. 1998. 'A Survey of Anonymous Oocyte Donors: Demographics', *Human Reproduction* 13(10): 2762–66.

Karlsen, S., L. Becares and M. Roth. 2012. 'Understanding the Influence of Ethnicity on Health', in G. Craig, K. Atkin, S. Chattoo and R. Flynn (eds), *Understanding 'Race' and Ethnicity: Theory, History, Policy, Practice*. London: Policy Press, pp. 115–32.

Kaufman, E. 2010. *Shall the Religious Inherit the Earth?* Exmouth: Profile Books.

Kazem, R., L.A. Thompson, M.P.R. Hamilton and A.Templeton. 1995. 'Current Attitudes towards Egg Donation among Men and Women', *Human Reproduction* 10(6): 1543–48.

Khalaji, M. 2006. 'The Last Marja: Sistani and the End of Traditional Religious Authority in Shiism' (Policy Focus 59). Washington, DC: Washington Institute for Near East Policy.

Khamene'i, A. al-. 2006. Ajwibat al-istift ' t: Al-'ib d t wa-l-mu' mal t. Beirut: al-Dar al-Islamiyah.

Khanna, S.K., M. Cheyney and M. Engle. 2009. 'Cultural Competency in Health Care: Evaluating the Outcomes of a Cultural Competency Training among Health Care Professionals', *Journal of the National Medical Association* 101(9): 886–92.

Kielman, K. 1998. 'Barren Ground: Contesting Identities of Infertile Women in Pemba, Tanzania', in M. Lock and P.A. Kaufert (eds), *Pragmatic Women and Body Politics*. Cambridge: Cambridge University Press, pp 127–63.

Kim-Godwin, Y.S., P.N. Clarke and L. Barton. 2001. 'A Model for the Delivery of Culturally Competent Community Care', *Journal of Advanced Nursing* 35(6): 918–25.

Kleinman, A. 1992. 'Local Worlds of Suffering: An Interpersonal Focus for Ethnographies of Illness Experience', *Qualitative Health Research* 2: 127–34.

———. 1997. *Writing at the Margins: Discourse between Anthropology and Medicine*. Berkeley: University of California Press.

———. 2006. *What Really Matters: Living a Moral Life amidst Uncertainty and Danger*. New York: Oxford University Press.

Knecht, M., M. Klotz and S. Beck. 2012. *Reproductive Technologies as Global Form*. Chicago: Campus Press and University of Chicago Press.

Knott, K. 1991. 'Bound to Change? The Religions of South Asians in Britain', in S. Vertovec (ed.), *Aspects of the South Asian Diaspora*. New Delhi: Oxford University Press, pp. 86–111.

Kroløkke, C. 2012. 'From India With Love: Troublesome Citizens of Fertility Travel', *Cultural Politics* 8(2): 307–25.

Kuku, S.F., and N.D. Osegbe. 1989. 'Oligo/Azoospermia in Nigeria', *Archives of Andrology* 22(3): 233–37.

Kumar, K. 2008. 'Core Ethnicities and the Problem of Multiculturalism: The British Case', in J. Eade, M. Barrett, C. Flood and R. Race (eds), *Advancing Multiculturalism, Post 7/7*. Newcastle: Cambridge Scholars Publishing, pp. 116–34.

Laidlaw, James. 2002. 'For an Anthropology of Ethics and Freedom', *Journal of the Royal Anthropological Institute* 8(2): 311–32.

Lambert, H. 2001. 'Not Talking About Sex in India: Indirection and the Communication of Bodily Intention', in J. Hendry and C.W. Watson (eds), *An Anthropology of Indirect Communication*. London and New York: Routledge, pp. 51–67.

Law, I. 2003. *Race, Ethnicity and Social Policy*. Hemel Hempstead: Prentice Hall.

Leavitt, R.L. 2002. 'Developing Cultural Competence in a Multicultural World', *Magazine of Physical Therapy* 10(12): 36.

Leonard, L. 2002. 'Problematizing Fertility: "Scientific" Accounts and Chadian Women's Narratives: Infertility around the Globe', in M. Inhorn and F. Van Balen (eds), *Infertility around the Globe: New Thinking on Childlessness, Gender, and Reproductive Technologies*. Berkeley: University of California Press, pp. 193–214.

Lessor, R., K. Reitz, J. Balmaceda and R. Asch. 1990. 'A Survey of Public Attitudes toward Oocyte Donation between Sisters', *Human Reproduction* 5(7): 889–92.

Letherby, G. 1999. 'Other than Mother and Mothers as Others: The Experience of Motherhood and Non-Motherhood in Relation to "Infertility" and "Voluntary Childlessness"', *Women's Studies International Forum* 22(3): 359–72.

Levi-Strauss, C. 1996. *The Savage Mind*. Chicago: University of Chicago Press.

Lo, M.M., and C.L. Stacey. 2008. 'Beyond Cultural Competence: Bourdieu, Patients and Clinical Encounters', *Sociology of Health and Illness* 30(5): 741–55.

Lotfalian, M. 2004. *Islam, Technoscientific Identities, and the Culture of Curiosity*. Washington, DC: University Press of America.
Lui, S.C., and S.M. Weaver. 1996. 'Attitudes and Motives of Semen Donors and Non-Donors', *Human Reproduction* 11(9): 2061–66.
Lutz, W., and A. Goujon. 2001. 'The World's Changing Human Capital Stock: Multi-State Population Projections by Educational Attainment', *Population and Development Review* 27(3): 323–29.
Macklin, R.B. 1995. 'Reproductive Technologies in Developing Countries', *Bioethics* 9: 276–82.
Madge, V. 2011. 'Infertility, Women and Assisted Reproductive Technologies: An Exploratory Study in Pune, India', *Indian Journal of Gender Studies* 18(1): 1–26.
Malpani, A., and A. Malpani. 2002. 'Simplifying Assisted Conception Techniques to Make Them Universally Available: A View From India', *Human Reproduction* 7(1): 49–50.
Mehta, B., and S. Kapadia. 2008. 'Experiences of Childlessness in an Indian Context: A Gender Perspective', *Indian Journal of Gender Studies* 15(3): 437–60.
Meyer, C.L. 1997. *The Wandering Uterus: Politics and the Reproductive Rights of Women*. New York: New York University Press.
Ministry of Health. 2001. 'Botswana HIV/AIDS Impact Survey'. Retrieved on 1 May 2014 from http://www.gov.bw/Global/NACA%20Ministry/wana/BAIS%20III_Stats%20Press.pdf
———. 2004. 'Botswana HIV/AIDS Impact Survey II RESULTS'. Retrieved on 1 May 2014 from http://www.gov.bw/Global/NACA%20Ministry/wana/BAIS%20III_Stats%20Press.pdf
———. 2009. 'Botswana HIV/AIDS Impact Survey III RESULTS'. Retrieved on 1 May 2014 from http://www.gov.bw/Global/NACA%20Ministry/wana/BAIS%20III_Stats%20Press.pdf
Mir, G., A. Nocon and W. Ahmad, with L. Jones. 2001. *Learning Difficulties and Ethnicity*. London: Department of Health.
Mirza, H.M. 2010. 'Rethinking Race', *Prospect* (October): 31–32.
Modood, T. 1997. '"Difference", Cultural Racism and Anti-Racism', in P. Werbner and T. Modood (eds), *Debating Cultural Hybridity: Multicultural Identities and Politics of Anti-Racism*. London: Zed Books, pp. 154–72.
———. 2008. 'South Asian Assertiveness in Britain', in S. Koshy and R. Radhakrishnan (eds), *Transnational South Asians: The Making of Neo-Diaspora*. Oxford: Oxford University Press, pp. 124–45.
Mody, P. 2008. *The Intimate State: Love-Marriage and the Law in Delhi*. London, New York and New Delhi: Routledge.
Mukherjee, M., and S.B. Nadimipally. 2006. 'Assisted Reproductive Technologies in India', *Development* 49(4): 128–34.
Muller, C.A. 1999. *Rituals of Fertility and the Sacrifice of Desire: Nazarite Women's Performance in South Africa*. Chicago: University of Chicago Press.

Murage, A., M.C. Muteshi and F. Githae. 2011. 'Assisted Reproduction Services Provision in a Developing Country: Time to Act?', *Fertility and Sterility* 96(4): 966–68.

Nabaitu, J., C. Bachengana and J. Seeley. 1994. 'Marital Instability in a Rural Population in South-West Uganda: Implications for the Spread of HIV-1 Infection', *Africa* 64(2): 243–51.

Nachtigall, R.D. 2006. 'International Disparities in Access to Infertility Services', *Fertility and Sterility* 85(4): 871–75.

Nahar, P. 2010. 'Health-Seeking Behavior of Childless Women In Bangladesh: An Ethnographic Exploration', *Social Science & Medicine* 71(10): 1780–87.

———. 2012a. 'Link Between Infertility and Poverty: Evidence From Bangladesh', *Human Fertility* 15(1): 18–26.

———. 2012b. 'Invisible Women in Bangladesh: Stakeholders' Views on Infertility Services', *Facts, Views & Visions in ObGyn* 4(3): 149–56.

Nahar, P., and A. Richters. 2011. 'Suffering of Childless Women in Bangladesh: The Intersection of Social Identities of Gender and Class', *Anthropology & Medicine* 18(3): 327–38.

Nahar, P., A. Sharma, K. Sabin, L. Begum, S. Khaled Ahsan and A.H. Baqui. 2000. 'Living with Infertility: Experiences among Urban Slum Population in Bangladesh', *Reproductive Health Matters* 8(15): 33–44.

Nahar, P., and S. van der Geest. 2014. 'How Women in Bangladesh Confront the Stigma of Childlessness: Agency, Resilience, and Resistance', *Medical Anthropology Quarterly*, published online. DOI: 10.1111/maq.12094

Nahman, M. 2013. *Extractions: An Ethnography of Reproductive Tourism*. Houndmills: Palgrave Macmillan.

Nargund, G. 2009. 'Natural/Mild Assisted Reproductive Technologies: Reducing Cost and Increasing Safety', *Womens Health* 5: 359–60.

Nasr, S.H. 1994. *Ideals and Realities of Islam*. London: Aquarian Press.

National Institute for Health and Clinical Excellence (NICE). 2005. 'Improving Outcomes in Children and Young People with Cancer'. London.

Nature. 2006. 'Cheap IVF Needed' (editorial), *Nature* 442: 958.

Nazroo, J.Y. 2001. *Ethnicity, Class and Health*. London: PSI.

———. 2003. 'The Structuring of Ethnic Inequalities in Health: Economic Position, Racial Discrimination and Racism', *American Journal of Public Health* 93(2): 277–84.

Noorashikin, M., F.B. Ong, M.H. Omar, M.R. Zainul-Rashif, A.Z. Murad, A. Shamsir, M.A. Norsina, A. Nursahireen, N.S.M.N. Sharifah-The, and A.H. Fazilah. 2008. 'Affordable ART for Developing Countries: A Cost Benefit Comparison of Low-Dose Stimulation versus High-Dose GnRH Antagonist Protocol', *Journal of Assisted Reproduction and Genetics* 25: 297–303.

Oakley, A. 1981. 'Interviewing Women: A Contradiction in Terms', in H. Roberts (ed.), *Doing Feminist Research*. London: Routledge and Kegan Paul, pp. 30–61.

Ogle, S.M., et al. 2008. 'Sperm Banking for Adolescents with Cancer', *Journal of Paediatric Oncology Nursing* 25(2): 97–101.

Okonofua, F.E. 1996. 'The Case against New Reproductive Technologies in Developing Countries', *British Journal of Obstetrics and Gynaecology* 103(10): 957–62.

Okonofua, F.E., D. Harris and A. Odebiyi. 1997. 'The Social Meaning of Infertility in Southwest Nigeria', *Health Transition Review* 7(2): 205–20.

Okumu, C.V., R.K. Kamau and K.O. Rogo. 1990. 'Past Reproductive and Sexual Characteristics of Women with Tubal Infertility at Kenyatta National Hospital', *East African Medical Journal* 67(12): 864–72.

Ombelet, W. 2009. 'Reproductive Healthcare Systems Should Include Accessible Infertility Diagnosis and Treatment: An Important Challenge for Resource-Poor Countries', *International Journal of Gynecology and Obstetrics* 106(2): 168–71.

———. 2013. 'The Walking Egg Project: Universal Access to Infertility Care: From Dream to Reality', *Facts, Views & Visions in ObGyn* 5(2): 161–75.

———. 2014. 'Is Global Access to Infertility Care Realistic? The Walking Egg Project', *Reproductive Biomedicine Online* 28(3): 267–72.

Ombelet, W., and R. Campo. 2007. 'Affordable IVF for Developing Countries', *Reproductive Biomedicine Online* 15(3): 257–65.

Ombelet, W., I. Cooke, S. Dyer, G. Serour and P. Devroey. 2008a. 'Infertility and the Provision of Infertility Medical Services in Developing Countries', *Human Reproduction Update* 14(6): 605–21.

Ombelet, W., P. Devroey, L. Gianaroli and E. te Velde. 2008b. *Human Reproduction ESHRE Monographs* 1: 117.

Ombelet, W., and F. Van Balen (eds). 2010. 'Social Aspects of Accessible Infertility Care in Developing Countries', *Facts, Views & Visions in ObGyn. Issues in Obstretics, Gynecology and Reproductive Health*. Wetteren: Universa Press, pp. 66–72.

Ong, A., and S. Collier (eds). 2005. *Global Assemblages: Technology, Politics and Ethics as Global Problems*. Oxford: Blackwell Publishing.

Orobitg, G., and C. Salazar. 2005. 'The Gift of Motherhood: Egg Donation in a Barcelona Infertility Clinic', *Ethnos: Journal of Anthropology* 70(1): 31–52.

Ortner, S.B. 2006. *Anthropology and Social Theory: Culture, Power, and the Acting Subject*. Durham, NC: Duke University Press.

Palihawadana, T.S., D.M.A.B. Dissanayake, A. Harshani and P.S. Wijesinghe. 2012. 'Chlamydia Trachomatis Infection in an Infertile Population: A Cross-Sectional Study', *Sri Lanka Journal of Obstetrics and Gynaecology* 32(4): 85–88.

Palihawadana, T.S., P.S. Wijesinghe and H.R. Seneviratne. 2012. 'Aetiology of Infertility among Females Seeking Treatment at a Tertiary Care Hospital in Sri Lanka', *Ceylon Medical Journal* 57(2): 79–83.

Palloni, A., and H. Rafalimanana. 1997. 'The Effects of Infant Mortality on Fertility Revisited: Some New Evidence', CDE Working Paper No. 96–27. Madison, WI: University of Wisconsin-Madison.

Papastergiadis, N. 1997. 'Tracing Hybridity in Theory', in P. Werbner and T. Modood (eds), *Debating Cultural Hybridity: Multi-Cultural Identities and the Politics of Anti-Racism*. London: Zed Books, pp. 257–81.

Parkin, R., and L. Stone (eds). 2004. *Kinship and Family: An Anthropological Reader*. Oxford: Blackwell Publishing.

Penn, R., and P. Lambert. 2002. 'Attitudes towards Ideal Family Size of Different Ethnic/Nationality Groups in Great Britain, France and Germany', *Population Trends* 108: 49–58.

Pennings, G. 2002. 'Reproductive Tourism as Moral Pluralism in Motion', *Journal of Medical Ethics* 28(6): 337–41.

———. 2008. 'Ethical Issues of Infertility Treatment in Developing Countries', *ESHRE Monograph, Task Force on Developing Countries and Infertility* 1: 15–20.

Pennings, G., G. de Wert, F. Shenfield, J. Cohen, B. Tarlatzis and P. Devroey. 2009. 'ESHRE Task Force on Ethics and Law: Providing Infertility Treatment in Resource-Poor Countries', *Human Reproduction* 24(10): 1008–11.

Philippe, S. 2009. *Une Histoire de Bamako*. Brinin sur Sauldre: Grandvaux.

Phoenix, A. 2009. 'De-Colonising Practices: Negotiating Narratives from Racialised and Gendered Experiences of Education', *Race, Ethnicity and Education* 12(1): 101–14.

Pilcher, H. 2006. 'Fertility on a Shoestring', *Nature* 442(7): 975–77.

Plumner, K. 2003. *Intimate Citizenship: Private Decisions and Public Dialogues*. Seattle: University of Washington Press.

Purdie, A., J.C. Peek, V. Adair and F. Graham. 1994. 'Attitudes of Parents of Young Children to Sperm Donation Implications for Donor Recruitment', *Human Reproduction* 9(7): 1355–58.

Purewal, S., and O. van den Akker. 2006. 'British Women's Attitudes towards Oocyte Donation: Ethnic Differences and Altruism', *Patient Education and Counselling* 64(1–3): 43–49.

———. 2007. 'The Socio-cultural and Biological Meaning of Parenthood', *Journal of Psychosomatic Obstetrics and Gynecology* 28(2): 79–86.

———. 2009. 'Systematic Review of Oocyte Donation: Investigating Attitudes, Motivations and Experiences', *Human Reproduction Update* 15(5): 499–515.

Qiu, R. 2002 'The Tension between Biomedical Technology and Confucian Values', in Julia Lai Po-wah Tai (ed.), *Cross-Cultural Perpsective on the (Im)possibility of Global Bioethics*. Dordecht: Kluwer, pp. 71–88.

Qureshi, K., K. Charsley and A. Shaw. 2012. 'Marital Instability among British Pakistanis: Transnationality, Conjugalities and Islam', *Ethnic and Racial Studies* 37(2): 261–79.

Rabinow, P. 1996. 'Artificiality and Enlightenment: From Sociobiology to Biosociality', in P. Rabinow (ed.), *Essays on the Anthropology of Reason*. Princeton, NJ: Princeton University Press, pp. 91–111.

Ragone, H. 1994. *Surrogate Motherhood: Conception in the Heart*. Boulder, CO: Westview Press.

Rapp, R. 1988. 'Moral Pioneers: Women, Men and Fetuses on a Frontier of Reproductive Technology', in F. Amadeo, E. D'Adamo, E.H. Baruch and J. Seager (eds), *Embryos, Ethics, and Women's Rights: Exploring the New Reproductive Technologies*. New York: Haworth Press, pp. 101–16.

———. 1998. *Testing Women, Testing the Fetus: The Social Impact of Amniocentesis in America*. London: Routledge.

———. 2001. 'Gender, Body, Biomedicine: How some Feminist Concerns Dragged Reproduction to the Centre of Social Theory', *Medical Anthropology Quarterly* 15(4): 466–77.

Rashid, S.F., and K. Dristi. 2007. '"Stolen Babies" and "Blocked Uterus": Poverty and Infertility Anxieties among Married Adolescent Women Living in a Slum in Dhaka, Bangladesh', *Anthropology and Medicine* 14(2): 153–66.

Remennick, L. 2006. 'The Quest for the Perfect Baby: Why Do Israeli Women Seek Prenatal Genetic Testing?', *Sociology of Health and Illness* 28(1): 21–53.

Renate, K.D. 1989. *Infertility: Women Speak Out about their Experiences of Reproductive Medicine*. London: Pandora Press.

Riessman, C.K. 2000. 'Stigma and Everyday Resistance Practices: Childless Women in South India', *Gender and Society* 14(1): 111–35.

———. 2002. 'Positioning Gender Identity in Narratives of Infertility: South Indian Women's Lives in Context', in M.C. Inhorn and F. Van Balen (eds), *Infertility Around the Globe: New Thinking on Childlessness, Gender, and Reproductive Technologies*. Berkeley: University of California Press, pp. 33–51.

Rispler-Chaim, V. 1993. *Islamic Medical Ethics in the Twentieth Century*. Leiden: Brill.

Ritchie, J., and L. Spencer. 1994. 'Qualitative Data Analysis for Applied Policy Research', in A. Bryman and B. Burgess (eds), *Analysing Qualitative Data*. London: Routledge, pp. 173–94.

Rob, U., and M.U. Mutahara. 2001. 'Premarital Sex among Urban Adolescents. The Population Council, Dhaka, Bangladesh', *Quarterly of Community Health Education* 20(1): 103–11.

Roberts, E.F.S. 2006. 'God's Laboratory: Religious Rationalities and Modernity in Ecuadorian In-Vitro Fertilization', *Culture Medicine and Psychiatry* 30: 507–36.

———. 2009. 'The Traffic between Women: Female Alliance and Familial Egg Donation in Ecuador', in D. Birenbaum-Carmelli and M.C. Inhorn (eds), *Assisting Reproduction, Testing Genes: Global Encounters with New Biotechnologies*. New York and Oxford: Berghahn Books, pp. 113–43.

Rodin, D.A., G. Bano, J.M. Bland, K. Taylor and S.S. Nussey. 1998. 'Polycystic Ovaries and Associated Metabolic Abnormalities in Indian Subcontinent Asian Women', *Clinical Endocrinology* 49: 91–99.

Rose, N. 2007. *The Politics of Life Itself. Biomedicine, Power, and Subjectivity in the Twenty-First Century*. Princeton, NJ: Princeton University Press.

Rouse, C. 2009. *Uncertain Suffering: Racial Health Disparities and Sickle Cell Disease*. Berkeley: University of California Press.

Rowe, P.J. 1999. 'Clinical Aspects of Infertility and the Role of Healthcare Service', *Reproductive Health Matters* 7(13): 103–11.

Rowland, R. 1992. *Living Laboratories: Women and Reproductive Technology*. Melbourne: Pan Macmillan Publishers.

RCP, RCR and RCOG. 2007. 'The Effects of Cancer Treatment on Reproductive Functions: Guidance on Management'. Report of a working party of the Royal College of Physicians, Royal College of Radiologists and Royal College of Obstetricians and Gynaecologists. Retrieved on 14 March 2010 from http://bookshop.rcplondon.ac.uk/contents/8ebae30b-2975-4858-bf30-d6561ea4f62a.pdf

Rutstein, S.O., and H.S. Iqbal. 2004. *Infecundity, Infertility, and Childlessness in Developing Countries: Issue 9 of DHS Comparative Reports*. Geneva: World Health Organization; and ORC Macro.

Sachedina, A. 2009. *Islamic Biomedical Ethics: Principles and Application*. Oxford: Oxford University Press.

Sallam, H.N. 2008. 'Infertility in Developing Countries: Funding the Project', *Human Reproduction ESHRE Monographs*, pp. 97–101.

Sami, N., and T.S. Ali. 2006.'Health Seeking Behaviour of Couples With Secondary Infertility', *Journal of the College of Physicians and Surgeons – Pakistan* 16(4): 261–64.

Sandelowski, M. 1991. 'Compelled to Try: The Never-Enough Quality of Connective Technology', *Medical Anthropology Quarterly* 5(1): 29–47.

Sandelowski, M., and S. Lacey. 2002. 'The Uses of a Disease: Infertility as Rhetorical Vehicle', in M.C. Inhorn and F. Van Balen (eds), *Infertility around the Globe: New Thinking on Childlessness, Gender, and Reproductive Technologies*. Berkeley: University of California Press, pp. 33–51.

Saniei, M. 2012. 'Human Embryonic Stem Cell Research in Iran: The Significance of the Islamic Context', in M. Inhorn and S. Tremayne (eds), *Islam and Assisted Reproductive Technologies: Sunni and Shia Perspectives*. New York: Berghahn Books, pp. 194–217.

Sariola, S., and B. Simpson. 2011. 'Theorising the "Human Subject" in Biomedical Research: International Clinical Trials and Bioethics' Discourses in Contemporary Sri Lanka', *Social Science & Medicine* 73(4): 515–21.

Schapera, I. (1940) 1971. *Married Life in an African Tribe*. Harmondsworth: Penguin Books.

Scheppers, E., E. van Dongenb, J. Dekkerc, J. Geertzend and J. Dekkere. 2006. 'Potential Barriers to the Use of Health Services among Ethnic Minorities: A Review', *Family Practice* 233(3): 325–48.

Schütz, A. (1932) 1967. *The Phenomenology of the Social World*. Trans. G. Walsh and F. Lehnert. London and Edinburgh: Heinemann Educational Books Ltd.

Seneviratne, H.R. 2011. 'Ethical Issues in the Provision of Assisted Reproduction', *Sri Lanka Journal of Obstetrics & Gynaecology* 33(3): 77–83.

Seneviratne, H.R., D. Lankeshwara, S. Wijeratne, N. Somasunderan and D. Athukorale. 2009. 'Serum Insulin Patterns and the Relationship between Insulin Sensitivity and Glycaemic Profile in Women with Polycystic Syndrome', *BJOG: An International Journal of Obstetrics and Gynaecology* 116: 1722–28.

Serour, G.I. 1995. 'Bioethics in Medically Assisted Conception in the Muslim World', *Journal of Assisted Reproductive Genetics* 12: 559–65.

———. 2006. 'Religious Perspectives of Ethical Issues in ART. Contemporary Ethical Dilemmas', in F. Shenfield and C. Sureau (eds), *Assisted Reproduction*. London: Informa Healthcare, pp. 99–114.

Shaery-Eisenlohr, R. 2008. *Shi'ite Lebanon: Transnational Religion and the Making of Religious Identities*. New York: Columbia University Press.

Shahin, A.Y. 2007. 'The Problem of IVF Cost in Developing Countries: Has Natural Cycle IVF a Place?', *Reproductive Biomedicine Online* 15: 51–56.

Shanawani, H., and M.H. Khalil. 2008. 'Reporting on "Islamic Bioethics" in the Medical Literature: Where are The Experts?', in J. Brockopp and T. Eich (eds), *Muslim Medical Ethics: From Theory to Practice*. Columbia: University of South Carolina Press, pp. 213–28.

Sharma, S., S. Mittal and P. Aggarwal. 2009. 'Management of Infertility in Low-Resource Countries', *British Journal of Obstetrics and Gynaecology* 116 (Supp. 1): 77–83.

Shaw, A. 2000. *Kinship and Continuity: Pakistani Families in Britain*. Amsterdam: Harwood Academic Publishers.

———. 2001. 'Kinship, Cultural Preference and Immigration: Consanguineous Marriage among British Pakistanis', *Journal of the Royal Anthropological Institute* 7(1): 315–34.

———. 2009. *Negotiating Risk: British Pakistani Experiences of Genetics*. Oxford and New York: Berghahn Books.

———. 2011. 'Risk and Reproductive Decisions: British Pakistani Couples' Responses to Genetic Counseling', *Social Science & Medicine* 73(1): 111–20.

Shaw, A., and J.A. Hurst. 2009. '"I Don't See Any Point in Telling Them": Attitudes to Sharing Genetic Information in the Family and Carrier Testing of Relatives among British Pakistani Adults Referred to a Genetics Clinic', *Ethnicity and Health* 14(2): 205–24.

Sheikh, A., and A. Esmail. 2007. 'Should Muslims Have Faith Based Health Services?', *British Medical Journal* 334: 74–75.

Simpson, B. 2000. 'Imagined Genetic Communities: Ethnicity and Essentialism in the 21st Century', *Anthropology Today* 16(3): 3–6.

———. 2001a. 'Ethical Regulation and the New Reproductive Technologies in Sri Lanka: Perspectives of Ethics Committee Members', *Ceylon Medical Journal* 46(2): 54–57.

———. 2001b. 'Making "Bad" Deaths "Good"': The Kinship Consequences of Posthumous Conception', *Journal of the Royal Anthropological Institute* 7(1): 1–18.

Simpson, B. 2004a. 'Localising a brave new world: new reproductive technologies and the politics of fertility in contemporary Sri Lanka', in M. Unithan-Kumar (ed.) *Reproductive Agency, Medicine and the State*. New York/Oxford: Berghahn Books, pp. 43–58.

Simpson, B. 2004b. 'Gays, Paternity and Polyandry: Making Sense of New Family Forms in Contemporary Sri Lanka', in C. Osella, F. Osella and R. Chopra (eds) *South Asian Masculinities*. Delhi: Kali, pp.160–74.

Simpson, B, 2004c 'Acting Ethically, Responding Culturally: Framing the New Reproductive and Genetic Technologies in Sri Lanka' *The Asia Pacific Journal of Anthropology* 5(3): 227–243.

Simpson, B. 2005. 'Impossible gifts: Bodies, Buddhism and Bioethics in contemporary Sri Lanka', *Journal of Royal Anthropological Institute* 10 (4): 839–859.

Simpson, B. 2009. 'We Have Always Been Modern: Buddhism, Science and the New Genetic and Reproductive Technologies in Sri Lanka.' *Culture and Religion An Interdisciplinary Journal* 10(2): 137–57.

Simpson, B. 2012. 'Legacies and Linkages: Episodes in the Establishment of New Reproductive Technologies in Sri Lanka'. in M. Knecht, M., Beck, S. and M. Klotz. (eds) *Reproductive Technologies as Global Form*. Chicago: Campus Press and University of Chicago Press. Pp 61–80.

Simpson, B. 2013. 'Managing Potential in Arts: Reflections on Gifts, Kinship and the Process of Vernacularisation'. *Current Anthropology* 54(supplement 7):1–11.

Simpson, B., Dissanayake, V.H.W. and R.W. Jayasekara. 2005. 'Contemplating Choice: Attitudes Towards Intervening in Human Reproduction in Sri Lanka', *New Genetics and Society* 24:99–117.

Skoog Svanberg, A., C. Lampic, T. Bergh and Ö. Lundkvist. 2003. 'Public Opinion Regarding Oocyte Donation in Sweden', *Human Reproduction* 18(5): 1107–14.

Sobotka, T. 2008. 'The Rising Importance of Migrants for Childbearing in Europe'. *Demographic Research* 19: 225–247.

Sri Lanka Medical Council. 2005. *The Assisted Reproductive Technologies Guidelines Committee: A Provisional Code of Practice For Assisted Reproductive Technologies*. Colombo: Sri Lanka Medical Council.

Stekelenburg, J., Jager, B.E., Kolk P.R,. Westen, E.H,. van der Kwaak A and I.N. Wolffers. 2005. 'Health Care Seeking Behaviour and Utilization of Traditional Healers in Kalabo, Zambia', *Health Policy* 71(1):67–81.

Strathern, M. 1992a. *After Nature: English Kinship in the Late Twentieth Century*. Cambridge: Cambridge University Press.

Strathern, M. 1992b. *Reproducing the Future: Essay on Anthropology, Kinship and the New Reproductive Technologies*. Manchester: Manchester University Press.

Sundby, J. 1997. 'Infertility in the Gambia: Traditional and Modern Health Care', *Patient Education and Counseling* 31(1): 29–37.

Sundby, J. 2005. 'Infertility and Healthcare in Countries With Less Resources', in M.C. Inhorn, and F. van Balen, F. (eds), *Infertility Around the Globe: New Thinking on Childlessness, Gender, and Reproductive Technologies: A View From The Social Sciences*. Berkeley, CA: University of California Press, pp. 247–259.

Tappan, R. 2012. 'More than Fatwas: Ethical Decision Making in Iranian Fertility Clinics', in M. Inhorn and S. Tremayne (eds), *Islam and Assisted Reproductive Technologies: Sunni and Shia Perspectives*. New York: Berghahn Books, pp. 103–29.

Taylor, C. 1994. *Multiculturalism: Examining the Politics of Recognition*. Princeton: Princeton University Press.

Thapan, M. ed. 2005. *Transnational Migration and the Politics of Identity*. New Delhi: Sage.

Thewes, B., B. Meiser, J. Rickard and M. Friedlander. 2003. 'The Fertility and Menopause Related Needs of Younger Women With a Diagnosis of Breast Cancer: A Qualitative Study', *Psycho-Oncology* 12(5): 500–511.

Thompson C.M. 2002. 'Fertile Ground: Feminists Theorize Infertility', in M.C. Inhorn and F. van Balen (eds), *Infertility Around the Globe: New Thinking on Childlessness, Gender, and Reproductive Technologies*. Berkeley: University of California Press, pp. 52–78.

Thompson, C. M. 2005. *Making Parents: The Ontological Choreography of Reproductive Technologies*. Michigan: MIT Press.

Throsby, K. 2004. *When IVF Fails - Feminism, Infertility and the Negotiation of Normality*. Basingstoke: Palgrave Macmillan.

Tomlinson, M. and A.A. Pacey. 2003. 'Practical Aspects of Sperm Banking for Cancer Patients', *Human Fertility* 6(3): 100–105.

Tomlinson, M. J. Pooley, K. Pierce, A. and J. F. Hopkisson, 2010. 'Sperm Donor Recruitment Within an NHS Fertility Service Since the Removal of Anonymity', *Human Fertility* 13(3): 159–167.

Tremayne, S. 2006. 'Not All Muslims Are Luddites', *Anthropology Today* 22(93) 1–2.

Tremayne, S. 2009. 'Law, ethics, and donor technologies in Shia Iran', in M. Inhorn and D. Birenhaum-Carmeli (eds), *Assisting reproduction, testing genes: Global encounters with new biotechnologies*. Oxford: Berghahn Books, pp. 144–63.

———. 2012. 'The "Down Side" of Third Party Donation: Challenging the "Happy Family Rhetoric" in Iran', in M. Inhorn and S. Tremayne (eds), *Islam and Assisted Reproductive Technologies: Sunni and Shia Perspectives*. New York and Oxford: Berghahn Books, pp. 130–56.

Turney, L. 2011. 'The Denial of Paternity: Pregnancy as a Risk to the "Pure Relationship"', *Sociology* 45(6): 1110–25.

Umezulike, A.C., and E.R. Efetie. 2004. 'The Psychological Trauma of Infertility in Nigeria', *International Journal of Gynaecology and Obstetrics* 84(2): 178–80.

Unisa, S. 1999. 'Childlessness in Andhra Pradesh, India: Treatment Seeking and Consequences', *Reproductive Health Matters* 7(13): 54–64.

———. 2010. 'Infertility and Treatment Seeking in India: Findings from District Level Household Survey', *Facts, Views & Visions in ObGyn, Monograph*: 59–65.

United Nations. 2004. *United Nations International Conference on Population and Development, Cairo 2004*, Retrieved on 25 June 2014 from: www.un.org/esa/population/cpd/cpd2004/CPD37_Res2004-2.

———. 2007. *United Nations Department of Economic and Social Affairs, Population Division (2007). World Population Prospects: The 2006 Revision, Highlights*, Working Paper No. ESA/P/WP.202.

Unnithan, M. 2010a. 'Infertility and Assisted Reproductive Technologies (ARTs) in a Globalising India: Ethics, Medicalisation and Agency', *Asian Bioethics Review* 2(1): 3–18.

———. 2010b. 'Learning from Infertility: Gender, Health Inequities and Faith Healers in Women's Experiences of Disrupted Reproduction in Rajasthan', *South Asian History and Culture* 1(2): 315–27.

Unnithan-Kumar, M. 2009. 'Female Selective Abortion – Beyond Culture: Family Making and Gender Inequality in a Globalising India', *Journal of Culture, Health and Sexuality* 12(2): 153–66.

Upton, R.L. 2001. '"Infertility Makes You Invisible": Gender, Health and the Negotiation of Fertility in Northern Botswana', *Journal of Southern African Studies* 27(2): 349–62.

Urdapilleta, L., C. Chillik and D. Fernandez. 2001. 'Do Fertile and Infertile People Think Differently about Ovum Donation?' *Journal of Assisted Reproduction and Genetics* 18(1): 1–7.

Van Balen, F. 2008. 'Involuntary Childlessness: A Neglected Problem in Poor-Resource Areas', *ESHRE Monograph* 1: 25–28.

Van Balen, F., and H.M.W. Bos. 2009. 'The Social and Cultural Consequences of Being Childless in Poor-Resource Areas', *Facts, Views & Visions in ObGyn* 1(2): 106–21.

Van Balen, F., and T. Gerrits. 2001. 'Quality of Infertility Care in Poor-Resource Areas and the Introduction of New Reproductive Technologies', *Human Reproduction* 16(2): 215–19.

Van Balen, F., and M.C. Inhorn. 2002. 'Interpreting Infertility: A View from the Social Sciences', in M.C. Inhorn and F. Van Balen (eds), *Infertility around the Globe: New Thinking on Childlessness, Gender, and Reproductive Technologies*. Berkeley: University of California Press, pp. 3–33.

Van Blerkom, J., W. Ombelet, E. Klerkx, M. Jansen, M. Dhont, G. Nargund and R. Campo. 2014. 'First Births with Simplified Culture System for Clinical IVF and Embryo Transfer', *Reproductive Biomedicine Online* 28(3): 310–20.

Van Zandvoort, H., K. de Koning and T. Gerrits. 2001. 'Medical Infertility Care in Low-Income Countries: The Case for Concern in Policy and Practice', *Tropical Medicine and International Health* 6(7): 563–69.

Vayena, E., H.B. Peterson, D. Adamson and K.G. Nygren. 2009. 'Assisted Reproductive Technologies in Developing Countries: Are We Caring Yet?' *Fertility and Sterility* 92(2): 413–16.

Vayena, E., P.J. Rowe and P.D. Griffin. 2002. 'Current Practices and Controversies in Assisted Reproduction'. Report of a meeting on 'Medical, Ethical and Social Aspects of Assisted Reproduction', held at WHO Headquarters in Geneva, Switzerland.

Vayena, E., J.P. Rowe and H.B. Peterson. 2002. 'Assisted Reproductive Technology in Developing Countries: Why Should We Care?', *Fertility and Sterility* 78(1): 13–15.

Verberg, M.F., et al. 2009. 'Mild Ovarian Stimulation for IVF', *Human Reproduction Update* 15(1): 13–29.

Verhaak, L., C.M. Smeenk, J.M.J. Evers and A.W.M. Kremer. 2007. 'Women's Emotional Adjustment to IVF: A Systematic Review of 25 Years of Research', *Human Reproduction Update* 13(1): 27–36.

Wade, P. 2007. 'Race, Ethnicity and Nation: Perspectives from Kinship and Genetics', in P. Wade (ed.), *Race, Ethnicity and Nation: Perspectives from Kinship and Genetics*. Oxford: Berghahn Books, pp. 1–32.

Werbner, P. 1997. 'Introduction: The Dialectics of Cultural Hybridity', in P. Werbner and T. Modood (eds), *Debating Cultural Hybridity: Multicultural Identities and the Politics of Anti-Racism*. London and New Jersey: Zed Books, pp. 1–26.

Werbner, R. 2004. *Reasonable Radicals and Citizenship in Botswana: The Public Anthropology of Kalanga Elites*. Bloomington: Indiana University Press.

Westlander, G., P. Janson, U. Tägnfors and C. Bergh. 1998. 'Attitudes of Different Groups of Women in Sweden to Oocyte Donation and Oocyte Research', *Acta Obstetricia et Gynecologica Scandinavica* 77(3): 317–21.

Whittaker, A. 2009. 'Global Technologies and Transnational Reproduction in Thailand', *Asian Studies Review* 33(3): 319–32.

Widge, A. 2005. 'Seeking Conception: Experiences of Urban Indian Women with In Vitro Fertilisation', *Patient Education & Counselling* 59(3): 226–33.

Widge, A., and J. Cleland. 2009a. 'The Public Sector's Role in Infertility Management In India', *Health Policy Plan* 24: 108–15.

———. 2009b. 'Assisted Reproductive Technologies in India: The Views of Practitioners', *Human Fertility* 12(3): 144–52.

Wijesinghe, D. 2012. 'Socio-Demographic Determinants of Subfertility in Sri Lanka', Annual Research Symposium 2012: Converging Technologies and Sustainable Communities. Colombo, Sri Lanka: University of Colombo, p. 54.

Wijeyaratne, C.N., R.De A. Senviratne, S. Dahanayake, V., Kumarapeli, E. Palipane, N. Kuruppu, C. Yapa and A.H. Balen. 2011. 'Phenotype and Metabolic Profile of South Asian Women with Polycystic Ovary Syndrome (PCOS): Results of a Large Database from a Specialist Endocrine Clinic', *Human Reproduction* 26: 202–13.

Williams, C., J. Sandall, G. Lewando-Hundt, B. Heyman, K. Spencer and R. Grellier. 2005. 'Women as Moral Pioneers? Experiences of First Trimester Antenatal Screening', *Social Science & Medicine* 61(9): 1983–92.

Wilkerson, J., and R. Parkin (eds). 2012. *Modalities of Change: The Interface of Tradition and Modernity in East Asia*. New York and Oxford: Berghahn Books.

Woliver, L.R. (ed.). 2002. *The Political Geographies of Pregnancy*. Urbana, IL: The University of Illinois Press.

World Bank. 2014. *Mali Country Report*. Retrieved on 24 June 2014 from http://data.worldbank.org/country/mali

World Health Assembly. 2004. *World Health Assembly Adopts First Global Strategy on Reproductive Health and Resolution on Family and Health*. Retrieved on 25 June 2014 from www.who.int/mediacentre/releases/2004

World Health Organization (WHO). 1987. 'Infections, Pregnancies and Infertility: Perspectives on Prevention', *Fertility and Sterility* 47: 944–49.

———. 2002. *Task Force on Diagnosis and Treatment of Infertility, Infections, Pregnancy and Infertility*. Geneva.

———. 2014. *Mali Country Report*. Retrieved on 24 June 2014 from http://www.who.int/gho/countries/mli.pdf?ua=1

World Population Review (WPR). 2014. *World Population Review: Mali*. Retrieved on 24 June 2014 from http://worldpopulationreview.com/countries/mali-population/

Zallum, A.Q. 1997. 'Islamic Verdict on Cloning, Human Organ Transplantation, Abortion, Test-Tube Babies, Life Support Systems, Life and Death', in Hizb ut-Taher series. Dhaka: Hizb ut-Taher, pp. 144–52.

Zaman, S. 2005. *Broken Limbs, Broken Lives: Ethnography of a Hospital Ward in Bangladesh*. Amsterdam: Het Spinhuis.

Zegers-Hochschild, F., G.D. Adamson, J. de Mouzon, O. Ishihara, R. Mansour, K. Nygren, E. Sullivan and S. Vanderpoel. 2009. 'International Committee for Monitoring Assisted Reproductive Technology [ICMART] and the World Health Organization [WHO] revised Glossary of ART Terminology', *Fertility and Sterility* 92(5): 1520–24.

Zeh, P., H.K. Sandhu, A.M. Cannaby and J.A. Sturt. 2014. 'Cultural Barriers Impeding Ethnic Minority Groups from Accessing Effective Diabetes Care Services: A Systematic Review of Observational Studies', *Diversity and Equality in Health and Care* 11(1): 9–33(25).

Index